Springer Biographies

More information about this series at http://www.springer.com/series/13617

Conrad Keating

Kenneth Warren and the Great Neglected Diseases of Mankind Programme

The Transformation of Geographical Medicine in the US and Beyond

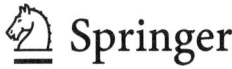 Springer

Conrad Keating
The Wellcome Unit for the History
   of Medicine
University of Oxford
Oxford
UK

ISSN 2365-0613   ISSN 2365-0621 (electronic)
Springer Biographies
ISBN 978-3-319-50145-1 ISBN 978-3-319-50147-5 (eBook)
DOI 10.1007/978-3-319-50147-5

Library of Congress Control Number: 2016960185

Cover Photo: Ken Warren Photo. Ken Warren circa 1979. Courtesy of Sylvia Warren.

Printed on acid-free paper

This Springer imprint is published by Springer Nature
The registered company is Springer International Publishing AG
The registered company address is: Gewerbestrasse 11, 6330 Cham, Switzerland

Foreword

This is the story of the life and work of a remarkable clinical scientist, Kenneth Warren. After describing Warren's early successes in medical research, mainly in the fields of parasitology, the story goes on to discuss his major achievement, which was the founding of a programme called the Great Neglected Diseases of Mankind. He achieved this by approaching leaders of research groups in several parts of the world, the work of which focused on diseases of the tropical belt. With the support of the Rockefeller Foundation, he offered financial help to each of the groups, and his only requirement was that they would meet together at least once each year to present their work to each other. In this way he was able to evolve valuable partnerships between workers in different but related fields. This remarkable programme lasted from 1978 to 1987 after which, sadly, it was terminated by the foundation.

There is no doubt that this programme had a very important effect on the evolution of research on many neglected diseases, particularly those of the tropical countries. Here is just one example: At the first and highly successful meeting of the chosen research groups in New York in 1978, there were several observers who were not related directly to the programme. One of them was Dr. Peter Williams, who at that time directed the Wellcome Trust in London, a medical research charity that later became one of the richest in the world. After the first day of the meeting was over, Dr. Williams invited me to his room and, stimulated by the day's programme, discussed how we could change the "field of tropical medicine" to "medicine in the tropics." In other words, how could partnerships be developed for research and capacity-building between rich and poor countries that not only would cover tropical disease but would also provide expertise and support in all aspects of medical research and care? The end result of this discussion was the development of highly successful partnerships between Oxford University and Thailand, Vietnam, and East Africa that are still fully active at the present time.

There is no doubt that although Kenneth Warren could be rather eccentric and difficult at times, his overall influence in developing ways to improve the health of poor countries, particularly those in the tropics, was extremely successful. It is a great pleasure to introduce this largely untold story while at the same time being able to thank Kenneth Warren and the Rockefeller Foundation for their personal support during the years of the Great Neglected Diseases of Mankind programme.

October 2015   Prof. Sir David J. Weatherall, MD, FRCP, FRS
                                                          Regius Professor of Medicine Emeritus
                                                     Weatherall Institute of Molecular Medicine
                                                        University of Oxford, Oxford, UK

Acknowledgement

This biography was supported by a grant from the Anthony Cerami and Ann Dunne Foundation for World Health, which is an independent institution devoted to sponsoring leading edge medical research, education and care. The commissioning fee and all subsequent royalties will be paid to The Wellcome Unit for the History of Medicine at the University of Oxford, in gratitude for their longstanding light-touch support and encouragement.

"One of the commitments of our foundation is to secure the stories of scientists whose defining purpose is to develop breakthrough solutions to human suffering. Ken Warren's contributions to the health of people in the developing world had been forgotten; we hope that this biography will help to underscore his role in helping to transform the global health agenda."

Ann Dunne

"This book is in memory of my dear friend Ken Warren, who gave me the courage to trust my scientific insights, and march against the consensus."

Anthony Cerami

Contents

About the Author

Conrad Keating is the Writer-in-Residence at the Wellcome Unit for the History of Medicine at the University of Oxford. He is the author of the widely-acclaimed biography of the British epidemiologist Sir Richard Doll, *Smoking Kills: The Revolutionary Life of Richard Doll.* His most recent publication, *Great Medical Discoveries: An Oxford Story*, accompanied the exhibition 'Great Medical Discoveries: 800 Years of Oxford Innovation' which he curated for the Bodleian Library. He lives in Oxford.

Introduction

In 1996, the dynamic medical researcher, Kenneth S. Warren, did a very rare thing: He spoke at his own memorial service.[1] In fact, the occasion was not a formal memorial event but rather the presentation of an honorary degree in recognition of his contributions to biomedical science and neglected tropical diseases. However, all of those in attendance, including Warren himself, knew that he did not have long to live. Perhaps, driven by the energy and scientific curiosity that were his lifeblood, he might well have echoed the sentiment of the physician William Osler, who in recognition of his own impending death, was heard to say, "I wish I could be there for the autopsy!"[2] The ceremony took place in June at the Picower Institute for Medical Research on Long Island, New York. Warren died of metastatic melanoma less than 3 months later on 18 September 1996.

Warren's career in medicine will be remembered for three enduring achievements: his efforts to introduce modern biomedical science to the study of infectious diseases in the developing world; the proselytising energy he brought to the ethical challenge of how to provide the most cost-effective health care to the world's poorest people; and his tenure as the Director of Medical Sciences at the Rockefeller Foundation (RF). Never short of grandiose ideas or audacious undertakings, Warren, while at the RF, played a pivotal role in shaping some of the most important campaigns to reduce the global burden of disease. His outstanding ability was his use of metrics to articulate health as an investment, not simply as expenditure. Furthermore, in the language of modern philanthropy, Warren had "convening power," which he used to mobilise powerful people, agencies, and institutions on behalf of the poor and the sick.

For Warren, and indeed for us all, life is lived with inevitable forward momentum, but very often the arc of its trajectory is only more properly understood in its final chapters. Certainly in Warren's case, much about his life scientific can be gleaned from the reactions to his death. In one of his obituary notices, he was

---

[1] Ann Dunne, personal communication.
[2] Bryant Boutwell, personal communication.

described in this unusual way: "Ken Warren has died. He was a boy of sixty-seven. I say 'boy' because he retained throughout his life all the enthusiasm and energy that he must have had at seventeen. If his body aged and was at last to betray him, his mind remained lively, sparkling, and faithful to the end."[3] The combination of boundless energy, intelligence, and being "inherently charismatic" enabled Warren to become a powerful force in global medicine in the second half of the twentieth century.[4] Even today, 20 years after his death, his contributions to the science of parasitology and the public-health strategies he championed are simultaneously lionised and questioned.

This equivocal perception can be better understood by recognising the polarising influence that Warren's personality and modus operandi had on his supporters and detractors. Warren was an iconoclast, yet he was both an establishment as well as a non-conformist figure. The celebrated immunologist, Michael Sela, encapsulates the anthropological paradox that Warren embodied: "[For me] with Ken it was love at first sight, because of his ideas and energy; but he was the most WASP-ish person I've ever met who had had a bar mitzvah!"[5] A driven, "larger than life character"[6] who had studied Literature at Harvard College "because he wanted to have subjects that he could talk to girls about,"[7] Warren developed a lifelong love of literature and poetry before going on to Harvard Medical School. Following the example of the British epidemiologist Jerry Morris, Warren was a devotee of the "three A's": analyst, agitator, and activist.[8] Possessing a contagious personality, he was full of charm and conviction, a straight-shooter who was allergic to concession and undeterred by confrontation. Equally, his ability to make friends as well as powerful adversaries began early. While a medical student at Harvard, and coming to the end of his studies, Warren sought career advice from Tom Weller, the virologist and Nobel laureate (Weller shared the Nobel Prize in 1954 for his work on poliomyelitis viruses). Receiving Weller's suggestion to go into public health and sanitation rather than tropical medicine, Warren took the opposite course, setting up years of future friction between the men.[9] Subsequently Warren and Weller were to take their disagreements over how to implement the most cost-effective form of medical treatment for infectious diseases into many public forums.

Outside of his immediate family, the closest person to Warren was Adel Mahmoud. A self-confessed "adopted son" of Ken and Sylvia Warren, Mahmoud forged his prodigious career under his mentor's influence and witnessed first-hand

---

[3]R. Selzer, "Obituary. Kenneth S. Warren, M.D. June 11, 1929–September 11, 1996". *Molecular Medicine,* Vol. 23, No. 6, November 1996.

[4]Don Bundy, personal communication.

[5]Michael Sela, personal communication.

[6]David Weatherall, personal communication.

[7]Adel Mahmoud, personal communication.

[8]Jerry Morris, personal communication.

[9]Adel Mahmoud, personal communication.

the polarising personality traits: "Early in his career Ken was widely respected as a scientist because he opened up the idea of mechanisms of disease in schistosomiasis. But his main stumbling block was his personality. If you could get along with him, you are in great shape. But if you're on the other side, and Ken is attacking you, and you're trying to attack him, you are going to have a hard time."[10] Others, such as Anthony Bryceson, who spent much of his life working on leishmaniasis in Africa, saw Warren as a man of quiet charm, who, while expecting people to go along with his ideas, would reward them with interest and praise.[11] Warren was certainly capable of being bombastic, eccentric, and swashbuckling, but these at-times-divisive components of his personality were tempered by the recognition in the minds of many that he had a great vision for tropical medicine and the delivery of health services in the tropics. On occasion, his enthusiasm sometimes bordered on the unrealistic, but the force of his will succeeded in carrying others with him. Warren's powers of persuasion were strengthened by the recognition, as noted by one of his colleagues, that "Ken was all heart. Above all he had the heart of an ox."[12] Physically, Warren was of average size, always well-dressed, hair groomed, very presentable but not showy—in the style of an American academic. The constants were a big smile and huge glasses.[13] He would walk very quickly and always had a full schedule of meetings to which he was hurrying, talking all the while about new ideas and possibilities.[14] He was fun to be with; not overly jovial but upbeat and animated.[15] In the words of his wife, Sylvia, "Enthusiastic was probably the best way to describe him. Very focused, very sure of what he wanted to do, and very adept at finding the best way to do it."[16]

The constant leitmotif running through Warren's work, and which, it could be argued, provided an apologia for his tendentious stance, was his dedication to the field of parasitology and to the poor people of the world whose lives were blighted by infectious diseases. For him, taking the numerical view of global health, substituting emotion with metrics, and achieving good health care at low cost would be achieved by the application of medical statistics and epidemiology, which he unsentimentally described as "medicine with the tears wiped off."[17] Warren was a man of science, and he knew that he ought to have no wishes or affections but instead a Darwinian heart of stone. Nevertheless, his own conversion to thinking globally about disease control came as an epiphany: "I was driving on a back road

---

[10]Adel Mahmoud, personal communication.

[11]Anthony Bryceson, personal communication.

[12]Gus Nossal, personal communication.

[13]Anthony Bryceson, personal communication.

[14]Julia Walsh, personal communication.

[15]Howard Klein, personal communication.

[16]Sylvia Warren, personal communication.

[17]K. S. Warren, "The Alma-Ata Declaration: Health for All by the Year 2000?", *Britannica Book of the Year*, *Encyclopedia Britannica*, Chicago, 1988. From a collection of Warren's private papers, p. 21.

in the Rift Valley of Kenya when I passed a large, apparently unruly crowd of Maasai who were attempting to wave me down. My first impulse was to put my foot on the accelerator, but in my rear view mirror I noticed what appeared to be several limp children in their arms. I turned back, and five men and women carrying four unconscious children jumped into the car while others tried to force their way in as well. As we drove frantically to the nearest aid station, about eight kilometres away, the adults moaned and cried while taking mouthfuls of cow's blood and milk from their gourds and blowing it on the children and all over the interior of the car. I don't think I've ever felt such a concentrated message of despair as those people evinced. Receiving that message, I suddenly realised how hardened I had become to the deaths of infants and children in the less developed world, and how I had assumed that the high death rates similarly inured parents to loss … Each day, tens of thousands of children die in the world's less developed countries for lack of adequate health care."[18] The experience was transforming for Warren: He felt very strongly that the deaths of children in poor countries mattered just as much as the deaths of children in rich countries and were a lot easier to prevent. For Warren, everyone scored the same in terms of importance.[19] He had identified a concrete problem, and he sought a scientific mechanism for its alleviation.

His ambitious plan was to create a scientific programme that would harness the new biological sciences to help alleviate the old parasitic diseases indigenous to the developing world. The idea had been incubating in Warren's mind for some time and was a direct result of his own laboratory work, much of which was undertaken at Case Western Reserve University (Cleveland, OH, USA) and had established his status as a renowned investigator in schistosomiasis.[20] This work was an early attempt to apply modern biomedical technology to the understanding of the mechanisms of disease prevalent in developing countries. With more than 3 billion people in those countries suffering from infectious diseases, Warren set himself the objective of finding the most cost-effective form of medical intervention to help reduce the sequence of "exposure, disability and death."[21] He was particularly interested in diarrheal and respiratory diseases (the biggest killers of children), neonatal death, and the delivery of vaccines. His path in life was set. The eminent Australian research immunologist, Gustav "Gus" Nossal, first met Warren in 1976 and was impressed by his ambitious vision: "His passion was to bring the fruits of the new biology, genetics and molecular biology to bear on tropical diseases,

---

[18]K. S. Warren, "The Alma-Ata Declaration: Health for All by the Year 2000?", *Britannica Book of the Year*, *Encyclopedia Britannica*, Chicago, 1988. From a collection of Warren's private papers, pp. 21–30.

[19]Richard Peto, personal communication.

[20]K. S. Warren, "Pathophysiology and pathogenesis of hepatosplenic schistosomiasis mansoni." Bull. N.Y. Acad. Med. 44: 280–294, 1968.

[21]J. A. Walsh & K. S. Warren, "Selective primary health care: an interim strategy for disease control in developing countries". *N. Engl. J. Med.* 301: 967–74, 1979.

which had been the domain of the older generation who had been out in Africa for twenty years, divorced from the new biology."[22]

Warren's vision was to establish a network of laboratories that would apply this "new biology" to the parasitic diseases prevalent in the developing world, particularly malaria and schistosomiasis. The opportunity for him to realise his global ambition came in 1977. Warren resigned from Case Western Reserve, where he had taught both in the medical school and in library sciences, and took up the post of Director of Health Sciences at the Rockefeller Foundation. Established in 1913, the Rockefeller charter states a noble objective: "to promote the well-being of mankind throughout the world." It was at the RF that Ken Warren forged his reputation for propagating the importance of scientific research to human well-being, and in so doing, made an enduring contribution to the transformation of disease control and global health. In December 1977, the RF Board of Trustees agreed, at Warren's suggestion, to establish the Great Neglected Diseases of Mankind (GND) programme, a project that would create "a network of high-quality investigators who would constitute a critical mass in this field, attract the brightest students and conduct research of excellence."[23] The idea was to bring together several research groups working on the more basic aspects of diseases of the developing world. The great neglected diseases were described as "great" in terms of prevalence and "neglected" in terms of the involvement of major international scientists and financial support. Warren, now with the financial backing of the RF, was going to roll out his synthesised programme, which would target diarrheal and respiratory diseases, malaria, schistosomiasis, African sleeping sickness, hookworm, and many other infectious diseases. The programme affirmed one of Warren's sacrosanct beliefs, i.e., that "a significant part of the investigator's efforts would be spent in applied collaborative research with colleagues in developing countries."[24] In this sense, the project would establish global networks that would link what he termed from "the bench to the bush."

The GND marked the fulfillment of an audacious undertaking to bring new biomolecular scientists to the field of parasitology, to create intellectual and personal connections between the different units, and to mould them into a strike force that was greater than the sum of its parts. This created an excitement about the science and a truly collaborative spirit. Keith McAdam joined the GND as part of Sheldon Wolff's team at Tufts University School of Medicine, and was immediately conscious of the scientific and social cohesion of the GND family: "Everyone had to go to the annual meeting, which helped to forge the GND into a major force that identified with the subject of parasitology, with Ken Warren and with the

---

[22]Gus Nossal, personal communication.

[23]K. S. Warren & C. C. Jimenez (eds), *The Great Neglected Diseases of Mankind Biomedical Research Network: 1978–1988.* New York: The Rockefeller Foundation, 1988, p. 1.

[24]K. S. Warren & C. C. Jimenez (eds), *The Great Neglected Diseases of Mankind Biomedical Research Network: 1978–1988.* New York: The Rockefeller Foundation, 1988, p. 1.

RF."[25] The programme also played a role in expanding the horizons of parasitology by funding a talented group of young researchers who reinvigorated the status of tropical medicine in the United States. A brilliant cohort of scientists—including John David, Adel Mahmoud, Anthony Cerami, James Kazura, Richard Guerrant, and Gerald Keusch—was persuaded by Warren to work on tropical diseases; otherwise, they might not have done so. Furthermore, the network brought research, education, and studies of diseases of the developing world to the mainstream of medicine in developed countries. Carlos Gitler, of the Weizmann Institute of Science in Israel, attended the inaugural meeting of the GND at Rockefeller University and was persuaded to transfer his research efforts to the understanding of diseases caused by parasites. At that meeting, held at the Abby Aldrich Rockefeller Hall in 1978, Gitler heard for the first time the famous Warren dictum: "Helminths are different from all other parasites in that they do not multiply in the host."[26]

Warren was a catalyser; his expertly delineated exhortations described how molecular science had the capacity to improve the human condition anywhere in the world, even in areas of great poverty at the edge of development. In many ways, this vision was prescient in that it took the study of neglected tropical diseases (NTDs) into the modern scientific age, and the network itself was very much a forerunner of contemporary disease-control practice. According to one of Warren's colleagues at the foundation, "Ken was an entrepreneur and an impresario. He was good at moving pieces around. He left his fingerprints all over that programme. He lived and breathed it."[27]

The GND Programme brought a stellar cohort into the field of parasitology, and their contributions to understanding the mechanisms of disease, improving human health, and transforming health outcomes are still relevant today. Warren's work has, according to his former colleague, Julia Walsh, "saved millions of children's lives."[28] His enduring role, according to Walsh, stems from their controversial study, "Selective Primary Health Care: An Interim Strategy for Disease Control in Developing Countries" (SPHC).[29] The paper advocated, contrary to the WHO view of total primary health care, a new turn toward selective and achievable goals by way of targeted assaults on specific diseases as implemented by the GND network. This approach had an enormous impact on health policy. For the first time, a study listed the diseases people died of so as to identify the biggest killers. It established a metric that could be used by donors, governments, and bilateral agencies for measuring the impact of the programme. It asked the fundamental question, "Is the programme that you plan to implement going to improve health in any way?"

---

[25]Keith McAdam, personal communication.

[26]C. Gitler in K. S. Warren & C. C. Jimenez (eds), *The Great Neglected Diseases of Mankind Biomedical Research Network: 1978–1988.* New York: The Rockefeller Foundation, 1988, p. 75.

[27]Joyce Moock, personal communication.

[28]Julia Walsh, personal communication.

[29]J. A. Walsh & K. S. Warren, "Selective primary health care: an interim strategy for disease control in developing countries". *N. Engl. J. Med.* 301: 967–74, 1979.

Within a couple of years, USAID declared that it would focus on child survival and implementing the policies of immunisations, oral rehydration, and breast feeding in line with the SPHC thinking described in the article by Warren and Walsh.[30] The policy's influence has been so far-reaching that "it massively changed the investment and resource allocation at UNICEF, at the WHO, USAID, [and] the World Bank."[31]

Ken Warren was a passionate communicator, a scientist with a feel for language, who embraced new technology as a way to get scientific information to make a difference. One of his favourite places in New York was The Century Association, a club for artists and amateurs in the arts, where he would hold post-work meetings to develop new programme ideas.[32] He was a friend and benefactor of the physician and writer Lewis Thomas, and Thomas's final collection of essays, *The Fragile Species*, was edited and published at Scribner under Warren's supervision. The art and practice of writing was close to Warren's heart, particularly because among his many fervently held ambitions had been to find ways for health workers in the developing world to have access to the most up-to-date biomedical knowledge. While at high school, Warren became fascinated by prose and poetry, and at Harvard, where he read American History and Literature, this developed into a love of books and writing.[33] His ambition to write may have been given metaphysical affirmation when, as a student at Harvard Medical School in the early 1950s, he double-dated with a friend, Richard "Dick" Norton, whose date was Sylvia Plath.[34] Dick and Ken were at Harvard Medical School together, but Dick didn't have a car, and Ken offered to drive him to Smith College in Northampton, Massachusetts, where Sylvia Plath studied, on the condition that he could be part of a double date. It is widely acknowledged that Dick Norton influenced the character of Buddy Willard in Plath's book, *The Bell Jar*, which was published in 1963.

Warren's creative energy aligned to an enviable command of the English language, which enabled him, according to his co-author Adel Mahmoud, "to write incredibly well."[35] In a professional career that spanned three decades, Warren wrote hundreds of scientific papers, numerous book chapters, 14 books, and, in 1994, he co-founded the journal *Molecular Medicine*, after a lifetime dedicated to expanding the frontiers of tropical and geographical medicine.

In many ways, Warren perfectly embodied the characteristics described by Isaiah Berlin in his 1953 essay, *The Hedgehog and the Fox*. In it the philosopher divided writers and thinkers into two categories: hedgehogs, who know one thing, and foxes who have many interests. Tellingly, in 1996, reflecting on his own personality and

---

[30]Julia Walsh, personal communication.

[31]Julia Walsh, personal communication.

[32]John Bruer, personal communication.

[33]R. Selzer, "Kenneth S. Warren" (obituary), *Molecular Medicine*, Vol. 2, No. 6, November 1996.

[34]Howard Klein, personal communication.

[35]Adel Mahmoud, personal communication.

style, Warren wrote: "I am broad-band multi-media digital broadcasting, constantly interrupting and bringing up new ideas and subjects... a constant stream of new ideas and schemes on everything."[36] Warren was most definitely a fox. Not content with his own research and the GND network, Warren's later career saw him help spearhead one of the most important experiments ever undertaken in world health.[37] In March 1984, at the RF's Bellagio lakeside retreat, a campaign was launched to immunise the world's children against six killer diseases (measles, tetanus, whooping cough, tuberculosis, polio, and diphtheria) in more than 100 countries before 1990. Meanwhile, he also pioneered new methods of electronic communication and the development of information science, increasing access to scientific journals, and sitting on the board of SatelLife, an organisation dedicated to linking health workers across the globe.

By advocating targeted assaults on specific diseases, Warren's approach continues to have enormous impact on health policy and health outcomes. His work and creative leadership have influenced researchers to think in more global terms about disease control, and his ideas continue to shape our world today. By any standard of measurement, this is a legacy deserving of greater examination and understanding.

---

[36]K. S. Warren, Speech given on 19 June 1996, Picower Institute for Medical Research. Courtesy of Sylvia Warren.

[37]June Goodfield, personal communication.

Chapter 1
The Rise

In science, or indeed in any field of endeavour, it is valuable to try and chart the timeline of an individual's interest in the subject that would redirect and dominate their life. Interestingly, for that generation of scientists born in the 1920s and 1930s, a book that is sometimes cited as first stimulating an interest in science is Paul De Kruif's *Microbe Hunters*, an easy-to-read book aimed at precocious high school students, which told the fascinating story of the microscopic life forms responsible for much human disease and the scientists who worked to end the suffering that they caused.

For Ken Warren, it was post–high school education that was to prove the formative influence on his future career in medicine. In 1950, the summer meeting of the US National Student Association was held at the University of Michigan. Warren attended the meeting as a representative of Harvard College. Also in attendance, representing Yale, was Scott Halstead. It was to prove a prophetic coincidence: Both men would go on to make valuable contributions to international health and also to work as colleagues at the RF 30 years later. Warren didn't enter Harvard Medical School until 1951, and it was not until he was well advanced in his medical studies that he decided to make his career in parasitology, but he knew that he wanted to travel and engage with the world. For Halstead, destiny was predetermined—his family background had been shaped by missionary work in China and India—and he came to international health from the prospective of a missionary's son "wanting to get out there and do something."[1] What the meeting in Michigan showed was that both men were activists by nature and were at ease representing and championing the rights of others.

Warren became a bibliophile while at Harvard College, where he majored in American History and Literature. His honours thesis considered the question of the poet T.S. Eliot's move to England from the United States in 1914. Showing the confidence and daring that were to be the hallmarks of his research techniques, he wrote to Eliot seeking an explanation. Warren's college roommate, C. Leonard

---

[1]Scott Halstead, personal communication.

© Springer International Publishing AG 2017
C. Keating, *Kenneth Warren and the Great Neglected Diseases of Mankind Programme*, Springer Biographies,
DOI 10.1007/978-3-319-50147-5_1

Gordon, recalled that "Eliot replied in a charming letter that he didn't feel he left America. He just found himself in England."[2] And whereas it was true that Warren wanted to have subjects that he could talk to girls about, there was also a curiosity and a need to satisfy his own psychological needs through the world of literature and the intellectual freedom it afforded him.[3] Warren knew that he wanted to study medicine, but he also recognised that literature was an essential guide to the psychology of healing. Although professional education could provide expert scientific training, it was literature that would prepare physicians to recognise and respond appropriately to all of the facets of human nature. Warren graduated cum laude from Harvard in 1951 and entered Harvard Medical School full of the energy and idealism that characterised his career. As a former roommate noted, "Ken not only knew that he wanted to be a doctor, he knew he wanted to explore the world, and he had a pith helmet ready to go."[4]

Early on in his training, Warren entertained the thought of becoming a paediatrician, but he ultimately decided that it would be too emotionally distressing. Instead, having resolved that the conventional practice of medicine was not for him and that tropical medicine was, he sought the advice of Tom Weller, the Nobel Laureate and Professor of Tropical Public Health at Harvard Medical School. The meeting did not go well, and rather than offering the advice that Warren wanted to hear, Weller told him to go into public health and sanitation. This marked the beginning of an enduring disagreement between the two men that was never resolved. However, their interests in natural history and helminthology were shared, and Weller had worked on the schistosome trematodes that cause schistosomiasis in humans, the parasitic disease that Warren would go on to spend almost his entire scientific career investigating. Schistosomiasis is a snail-borne infection, which in the early 1960s was estimated to afflict more then 150 million people worldwide. The genus Schistosoma includes several of the oldest human parasites known: *Schistosomiasis haematobium* eggs were found in the kidney of 20th-dynasty Egyptian mummies (1250–1000 B.C.). The urinary tract or the intestines may be infected. Signs and symptoms may include abdominal pain, diarrhoea, bloody stool, or blood in the urine. Those who have been infected a long time may experience liver damage, kidney failure, infertility, or bladder cancer. In children, it may cause poor growth or learning difficulties. It ranked second only to malaria in worldwide importance and was the subject of renewed scientific interest due to the proliferation of irrigation schemes and dams that were causing the disease to spread into areas where it had not previously been known.

In 1956, after his internship at Boston City Hospital, Warren joined the Laboratory of Tropical Diseases at the National Institutes of Health (NIH). During that period, Warren initiated the first detailed study of *Schistosoma mansoni* in mice describing the animal model and its relevance to the pathophysiology of the disease

---

[2]Nick Ravo, *The New York Times,* 19 September 1996.

[3]Adel Mahmoud, personal communication.

[4]Nick Ravo, *The New York Times,* 19 September 1996.

in humans.[5] There was a heavy emphasis on basic science in Warren's own research work, which was to be a major influence on the development of his ideas to provide new means of treatment and prevention of the great tropical and geographical diseases. He was probably the only physician in the Laboratory of Tropical Diseases, which later amalgamated with malaria research to become the Laboratory of Parasitic Diseases in 1960. He was interested in schistosomiasis, which offered an excellent prism through which to understand the science of parasitology. This fascination with schistosomiasis arose from two specific sources. First, on Warren's arrival in Bethesda, the director, Dr, Willard Wright, suggested that he "wonder about and pick a parasite."[6] Second, as an intern at Boston City Hospital, he had seen a large number of patients with alcoholic liver disease and was intrigued by the liver's involvement in schistosomiasis. Moreover, his imagination was captured when he saw *S*. mansoni–infected mice being studied by his colleague, Dr. William B. "Bill" DeWitt, who was interested in the effects of malnutrition on infection. Warren's early laboratory research concentrated on the quantitative aspects of the study of schistosomiasis, particularly worm numbers through perfusion of the portal system, and the counting of hepatic eggs in pepsin-digested liver fragments.[7] Following the maxim "seek out the ways of nature by experiment," coined by the great 17th-century medical investigator William Harvey, Warren had used his laboratory experience to refine his thinking.

Although the NIH had succeeded in expanding his scientific universe, Warren rarely stopped contemplating how to exact more effort, speed, and impact from his work. Accordingly, to pursue his interest in liver disease and to gain greater experience of treating people with tropical diseases, Warren went to London in 1958 to study for a Postgraduate Diploma in Tropical Medicine and Hygiene at the London School of Hygiene and Tropical Medicine (LSHTM). The institution was founded in 1899 by Sir Patrick Manson as the London School of Medicine and moved to its present location in Keppel Street in 1929. The purchase of the site and the cost of the building were made possible by the generous gift of $2 million by the RF. It seemed that from early on, Warren's medical interests and the RF's humanitarian cthos formcd a gcnuinc symbiosis. Thc Diploma in Tropical Mcdicinc and Hygiene was also particularly well suited for physicians who had trained in medicine in a developed country and intended to practice in the tropics. This was the career trajectory that excited Warren the most, and London had the added attraction of allowing him to pursue his interest in liver disease with the hepatologist, Professor (later Dame) Sheila Sherlock (1918–2001).[8] A formidably

---

[5]K. S. Warren & W. B. De Witt, "Esophageal varices in mice infected with *S. mansoni*." Proc. VI Internat. Cong. Trop. Med. & Malaria, Lisbon. 2: 115–119, 1958.

[6]K. S. Warren, "The bench and the bush in tropical medicine." Am. J. Trop. Med. Hyg. 30: 1149–1158, 1981.

[7]Allen Cheever, personal communication.

[8]K. S. Warren, F. L. Iber, W. Dolle, & S. Sherlock, "Effect of alterations in blood pH on distribution of ammonia from blood to cerebrospinal fluid in patients in hepatic coma." J. Lab. Clin. Med. 56: 687–694, 1960.

intelligent medical researcher, Sherlock in the 1950s was conducting research into portal hypertension, hepatic encephalopathy, and ascites. In 1958, the year Warren arrived in London, Sherlock was appointed the first Professor of Medicine at the Royal Free Hospital School of Medicine. There she founded the liver research unit, and the department attracted leading researchers from around the world. Her work helped to establish hepatology as a medical specialty, and her professionalism and insights must have had a profound influence on Warren's noted "precise" laboratory research techniques.[9]

Although London was not yet "swinging," Warren was captivated by his new environment, and over the years he gained a reputation for being an Anglophile.[10] He drove an MGB, liked to drink single malt whisky, and would greet colleagues with the English idiom "Hello my dear boy." The catalyst for this love affair may have been Sylvia Rothwell, an attractive English woman he met through the Oxford–Harvard diaspora. Sylvia had not studied at Oxford, although her younger sister Pamela had, but she was educated, well-travelled, and resolutely independent. On leaving school, Sylvia was determined to make her career in the fabric and fashion industry. After studying at the Central School of Art and Design and gaining an Institute of Wool Secretariat B.A. from Leeds University, her resolve gained her an interview at *Liberties*, the heritage British fashion company. However, during the interview she was told that before she could work there, she "could do with a bit more training." This she duly did. Funded by a King George IV memorial fellowship, Sylvia studied a 1-year postgraduate course at the Rhode Island School of Design. As well as getting valuable training, Sylvia showed a true spirit of adventure by touring the country, mainly on Greyhound buses, visiting every state in the Union with the exception of Arkansas and Nebraska. But the experience proved far from seductive, because on arriving back in the United Kingdom Sylvia announced that she would "never live in the US, and never marry an American!"[11]

This was the implacable mind set that foreshadowed Ken and Sylvia's meeting in London in the winter of 1958. By then, Sylvia had established herself within London's fashion industry, working first for Marks & Spencer's wool-buying department (which required visiting the two European capitals of fashion, Paris and Milan, and then advising woollen mills in Britain on design and colour), and by 1958 she was working at Jaeger's head office not far from the London School of Hygiene. But how did their first meeting go? Was it love at first sight for Sylvia? "Not in my case, not at all. In fact I was a little off put and I know exactly why! He was brash. He was very persistent, but eventually, I thought, 'well for heaven's sake, let's have lunch'."[12] Sylvia's apprehension was confirmed when Ken was late for this first date. The inappropriateness of his behaviour, of perhaps not treating

[9]Charles "Chuck" Carpenter, personal communication.

[10]Gerald Keusch, personal communication.

[11]Sylvia Warren, personal communication.

[12]Sylvia Warren, personal communication.

people in the most respectful way, was to be something people noted in Warren's character, and it did not always serve him well. After excelling at Stuyvesant High School in New York as well as Harvard, he had a sense of self-worth and an absence of false modesty. He was enthusiastic, determined, and had a great deal to offer, and consciously or unconsciously he projected a sense of entitlement. However, on this occasion, as was to happen over the next four decades, luck and the quality of his research redeemed the situation. The venue that he had chosen for lunch was Wheeler's, Sylvia's favourite fish restaurant in London. From then on he became less brash in her eyes, and things developed rapidly. Both were age twenty-nine, and with Ken due to return to the US in February 1960, it appeared to both of them that it was a question of now or never.

Early in 1960, Ken's wedding proposal was accepted, and a marriage date of 14 February was set. The speed of events didn't allow sufficient time to read the banns of marriage, which should have occurred over 3 consecutive Sundays. Being a "man of action," Ken wrote to the Archbishop of Canterbury seeking a special wedding license, which was duly granted.[13] The magnificent scroll-like license, complete with wax seal, was delivered to Sylvia at Jaeger's head office in time for their marriage ceremony. Their best man was the medical missionary, W. B. "Beas" Rogers Beasley, whom Ken had met on the DTM&H course and who, after leaving London, worked with the Frontier Nursing Service in Hyden, Kentucky; he was also godfather to both Warren children, Christopher and Erica.[14] Remarkably, a few days after getting married, Professor Sherlock offered Warren a temporary job at the Hammersmith Hospital for 6 months, which allowed for a more relaxed transition into married life before leaving for the US in July 1960.

Another factor cementing Warren's affection for England and the LSHTM was his friendship with Sir Philip Manson-Bahr, a leading figure in tropical medicine. Manson-Bahr edited *Manson's Tropical Diseases* from the 7th edition in 1921 through the 15th edition in 1960. They met at a tropical medicine meeting held in Portugal in 1960 and continued their friendship in England. Warren had driven to the meeting in a new Porsche that he had collected from the factory in Stuttgart. On arrival, he was greeted by Ferdinand Porsche himself, who put the sports car through its paces in what must have been a surreal demonstration for the young doctor.[15] In subsequent years, the friendship between Warren and Sir Philip was sustained thanks to a geographic coincidence. Sylvia's father, the physicist Percy Rothwell, lived in Westerham in Kent, whereas Sir Philip's home was in the nearby rural idyll of Pootings.

---

[13]Sylvia Warren, personal communication.

[14]W. B. Rogers Beasley, *The Family Nurse: Guidelines for a programme to extend medial manpower in Appalachia.* 1968.

[15]The money for the Porsche came from a loan from Warren's grandparents. Although there can't have been many NIH Fellows driving German sports cars around Washington DC in the early 1960s, this glamorous status symbol was later taken from Warren when Sylvia crashed the car near their home in Silver Spring, Bethesda.

After his work in England, Warren returned to the NIH convinced that that he wanted to study schistosomiasis in humans. Until then, he had been a quintessential lab-man: He had not, as it were, "strode the jungles or the deserts," and so it was essential that he find a position in the tropics.[16] A further compulsion was the birth of a son, Christopher, in late 1960, and with little prospect of promotion or securing additional funding at the NIH, Warren sought salvation by translating laboratory science to the clinic, or in his own memorable words, "from the bench to the bush." Serendipitously, new investigations into the application of laboratory work were soon forthcoming: The idea of using chemotherapy to control manifestations of schistosomiasis started with a paper published by a Brazilian researcher in 1962.[17] Warren was to take this concept and develop it into the intervention that became targeted chemotherapy. Allen Cheever joined the Laboratory of Parasitic Diseases in 1960, after an internship and a year of pathology at Mt. Sinai Hospital in New York, and witnessed at first-hand Warren's style: "Ken was many things but never unenthusiastic and never modest, and he seemed to spend a lot of time in the hallways recruiting people to 'come, look at this!' He saw what he wanted and got it. Much of what he learned was filtered through Rodney Duvall, Bill DeWitt's technician, an extremely adept and intelligent person."[18] Warren learned quickly, and was soon on the way to expanding the field by the creative force of his original work, scientific insights, and published papers.[19] Although Ken was developing a burgeoning blueprint for what became known as "science-based development," Sylvia found it difficult to pursue her professional career in Washington, a city overwhelmingly comprised of lawyers and government officials. This disappointment was lessened by the joy of their son, Christopher, and her delight at Ken's NIH work and his determination to get ahead: "He was very focused, very sure of what he wanted to do, and very adept at finding the best way to do it."[20]

Such an opportunity came in the spring of 1962, when Warren took up a 2-year appointment as Visiting Professor of Medicine at the University of Bahia in Brazil. His objective was to initiate a research programme on the pathologic physiology of human hepatosplenic schistosomiasis.[21] Specifically, he wanted to conduct clinical studies of patients with such manifestations of schistosomiasis as anaemia and hepatic coma and the possible relationship between ammonia toxicity and coma. Warren was joined at the project in Bahia by his friend, Grady V. Bryant, a research technician in the Laboratory of Parasitic Diseases. The men were following in a strong tradition because for many years the Laboratory of Parasitic Diseases and its

[16]Anthony Bryceson, personal communication.

[17]N. Kloetzel, "Splenomegaly in schistosomiasis mansoni." Amer J Trop Med Hyg 11: 472–476, 1962.

[18]Allen Cheever, personal communication.

[19]K. S. Warren, "The influence of treatment on the development and course of murine hepato-splenic schistosomiasis mansoni." Trans. R. Soc. Trop. Med. Hyg. 56: 510–519, 1962.

[20]Sylvia Warren, personal communication.

[21]*The NIH Record,* Volume X1V, No. 11. 6 June 1962, p. 3.

antecedent, the Laboratory of Tropical Diseases, had maintained an active research programme in many aspects of schistosomiasis. Scientists at the laboratory had been instrumental in establishing the efficacy of sodium pentachlorophenate as a snail-killing agent. They had done considerable work on the relation of nutrition to the effectiveness of chemotherapeutic agents against the adult worms that cause the disease as well as on the pathology of the disease. Warren, for his part, wanted to conduct a series of investigations on individuals with varying clinical conditions caused by schistosomiasis, and he had the good fortune to work with Gilberto Rebouças at the Hospital das Clínicas in Bahia [now Hospital Universitario Professor Edgard Santos].[22] Gilberto was an outstanding physician who had spent 2 years in Boston and who, according to Allen Cheever, was not "bruised" by "Ken's ego and brash behaviour."[23] The idea of using chemotherapy to control manifestations of schistosomiasis was the hinge on which Warren's scientific contribution to tropical medicine turned as he developed and promoted the idea of targeted chemotherapy.[24] This work, early in his career, paved the way for the application of modern biochemistry and immunology to the study of helminthic infection. Unfortunately, although his professional life flourished, his 2-year appointment in Brazil ended in tragedy. Grady Bryant was killed in a road accident the day before he was due to return to the US. Warren collected his friend's body from the hospital and held Grady's hand throughout the long overnight journey back to Bahia.

Professionally, Warren now stood at a crossroads: After 8 years at the Laboratory of Tropical Diseases, he knew he had little hope of securing another post-doctoral position or additional funding, so it was imperative that he find a new post in academic medicine—and one that would provide some level of independence. Serendipitously, Dieter Cook Fraser, from Case Western Reserve University, was also in Bahia on a research visit and suggested that Warren should apply for the post of assistant physician in Cleveland, Ohio. His application was successful, and without returning to the NIH, Warren moved with his family to Cleveland in 1963 to join the faculty at Case Western Reserve University. During the following 14 years, Warren would open up the idea of mechanisms of diseases in schistosomiasis and become a major force in the field of parasitology and a scientific investigator ahead of his time.[25]

One of the most distinguished figures in parasitology, Dame Bridget Ogilvie, recognised Warren's contribution to medical science forged whilst at Case Western

---

[22]K. S. Warren & G. Reboucas, "Blood ammonia during bleeding from esophageal varices in patients with hapatosplenic schistosomiasis." N. Engl. J. Med. 271: 921–926, 1964; K. S. Warren, G. Reboucas & A. G. Baptista, "Ammonia metabolism and hepatic coma in hepatosplenic schistosomiasis. Patients studied before and after portacaval shunt." Ann. Int. Med. 62:1113–1133, 1965.

[23]Allen Cheever, personal communication.

[24]K. S. Warren & A. S. Weisberger, "The treatment of molluscan schistosomiasis mansoni with chloramphenicol." Am. J. Trop. Med. Hyg. 15: 342–350, 1966.

[25]Adel Mahmoud, personal communication.

Reserve. Ogilvie herself had earned a doctoral degree at the University of Cambridge for work on *Naippostrongylus brasiliensis*, and in 1963 she joined the British Medical Research Council's National Institute for Medical Research spending her career studying immune responses to intestinal worms. For more than a decade as the Director of the Wellcome Trust, Ogilvie occupied a position of great influence in the world of tropical medicine. She had first met Warren at a parasitology conference in Washington in the late 1960s and greatly respected his scientific work, which she viewed as being in the vanguard of American parasitology. In fact, she saw Warren "as a breath of fresh air, and someone who began to get the Americans to do serious science. He did really beautiful work in the 1960s on the immunological basis of what happens to the schistosome egg in tissue. Ken was the first American I met who was doing serious science, and he transformed things."[26] Whereas in Britain in the mid-1960s, Ogilvie and her colleagues were addressing one of the fundamental questions in parasitology: Why did some parasites escape the body's immune response? Thus, many leading figures in US parasitology—such as Elvio Sadun and Franz von Leichtenberg—continued to be mainly interested in descriptive science rather than attempting to analyse the immune response to parasites. Warren's innovative approach, e.g., examining T-cell–mediated pathology, represented an experimental advance and was an outlier to the realignment of the subspecialty in the US. He was interested in the what, why and how of the host–parasite relationship, essentially, the mechanism of disease in schistosomiasis.

To better understand the interplay between measuring the burden of schistosomiasis in developing countries and Warren's forceful role in championing the disease, it is important to place the story in its historical context. Although malaria is the most lethal parasitic disease of mankind, the World Health Organisation's (WHO) malaria-eradication programme had collapsed by 1970, and even in the 1960s it was obvious to many that there were fundamental shortcomings.[27] The disease was far from being eradicated, and between 1970 and 2000 the number of cases worldwide and the number of deaths steadily increased.[28] The rising death toll was primarily due to the increasing resistance of the *anopheline* vector to insecticides and of the parasite to the antimalarial drugs that were deployed. In fact, the feeling was that by 1970, the only place where malaria had been eradicated was in the mind of the WHO.

Into this malaise moved Dr. N. Ansari, Chief Medical Officer of the Division of Communicable Diseases at the WHO. Seeing the failure of the malaria programme, he quickly sought to introduce new directions and approaches to reinvigorate the division. Single-handedly, he pushed schistosomiasis higher up the health agenda, using the sophisticated political skills he had harnessed over years of working in

[26]Bridget Ogilvie, personal communication.

[27]David Bradley, personal communication.

[28]J. Farrar, P. J. Hotez, T. Junghanss, G. Kang, D. Lalloo, N. White (eds), *Manson's Tropical Diseases*, Twenty-Third Edition, p. 533.

international agencies. Ansari was widely respected, and—according to David Bradley, the former Ross Professor of Tropical Hygiene at the LSHTM who developed an epidemiological model of *S. haematobium*—"personified the ideal of an international civil servant; he did all the work, but didn't wave his name around."[29] In the mid-1960s, Bradley was in a unique position to see Ansari's bureaucratic maneuvering and clear thinking in operation. Bradley's boss, George Macdonald, Director of the Ross Institute of Tropical Medicine, was taken ill with what would be a fatal cancer, and Bradley, named as his substitute, found himself, only 2-years qualified in medicine, serving on the WHO Committee on Schistosomiasis. Bradley has spent much of his professional life working on the public-health importance of schistosomiasis and other water-related diseases and recognised the role that both Ansari and Warren played in showing the burden of schistosomiasis on the world's poor. Their respective methodologies differed greatly—Warren's hyperbole stood in stark contrast to Ansari's measured persuasion—but Bradley recognised that there was a shared goal, i.e., that of highlighting the plight of a neglected people. "Schistosomiasis was well established by Ansari, who pre-dated Ken Warren. They probably wouldn't have got on, as they had very different personalities; Ken had a very big ego and was pushing himself forward, whereas Ansari was diplomatic. But Ken wasn't an ungenerous person, and when he got into a position of power he did a good job."[30]

Another factor that drove concerns about the prevalence of the disease was the extensive dam-building programme of the period. The Aswan High Dam in Egypt and the Akosombo Dam in Ghana were among the vast new construction artificially enhancing the global freshwater snail habitat and increasing the local transmission of schistosomiasis. Two of the countries that experienced huge indigenous exposure to the disease were Egypt and Brazil, and the clinical experience that Warren gained in Bahia provided him with valuable insights into the pathology of the disease, which he built on in his work in Cleveland. From the outset, Warren's laboratory at the Institute of Pathology at Case Western Reserve became a powerhouse, launching the scientific careers of a cadre of researchers from the developing and developed world including Mohamed Farid Abdel-Wahab, Ernesto Domingo, Dov Boros, and Adel Mahmoud. Warren was a demanding taskmaster; he admitted to having an "intense scientific ambition," which necessitated working 6- to 7-day weeks, 12-hour days, and amassing academic papers in leading medical journals.[31] A prolific writer and researcher, Warren pushed himself, pushed at the future, and pushed the people who came within his gravitational pull. On meeting him for the first time, one was struck by his enthusiasm, charisma, and limitless energy—he was uneasy if he wasn't working, and his dedication to the cause, whatever that might be, was unswerving.

---

[29]David Bradley, personal communication.

[30]David Bradley, personal communication.

[31]Speech given by Ken Warren at the Picower Centre, 19 June 1996. Courtesy of Sylvia Warren.

In summer 1965, due to a sudden and unexpected financial hiatus, the research work being undertaken in his laboratory was endangered. The work had been supported by the Army Medical Research and Development Command on the recommendation of the Armed Forces Medical Board. Congress had cut the R&D Command's appropriation by 30%, which left a shortfall of $8000. In a letter to Dr. Gerard R. Pomerat, Associate Director of Medical and Natural Sciences at the RF, Warren balanced his application for funds with a justification for the continuance of the high-quality experimental programme. "Our attack on the problem of schisto-somiasis is proceeding along four lines: (1) The reproduction in the experimental animal of the various human disease syndromes associated with infection with *S. mansoni* and *Schistosoma japonicum*, and the elucidation of their pathogenesis. Specifically, we are studying clay pipestem fibrosis, intestinal lesion, anemia and cerebral lesions. (2) The individual host response to infection with schistosomes utilising quantitative counts of cercariae penetration, development of worms, egg output by worms and granuloma formation by the host. (3) Attempts to inhibit granuloma formation via immunosuppressive drugs in order to determine the role of the host response in the development of liver disease. (4) Suppression of schisto-somiasis in the snail (the formation of cercariae from miracidia) through the use of inhibitors of protein synthesis. We have achieved success in all of the above areas, and are entering into these problems in greater depth."[32]

Fortunately, something of a financial panacea arrived when Warren was appointed a career investigator of the NIH; as a consequence, he was assured of adequate research support for at least 5 years. Moreover, as Assistant Professor of Preventive Medicine and Tropical Medicine, he was the only parasitologist in the medical school and intertwined the subject in a course entitled, "Mechanisms of Disease." At the same time, his significant publications on basic research in schistosomiasis were getting him noticed,[33] and in May 1966, Virgil C. Scott, Associate Director of Medical and Natural Sciences at the RF made a site visit to Warren's laboratory. Scott was responsible for the RF's schistosomiasis field station on the island of St. Lucia in the Caribbean, and he was constantly looking to recruit young, hungry, and innovative research workers into the programme. Scott's diary, describing their first meeting at Case Western, offers an interesting portrait of the dynamic between benefactor and apprentice. "He has been at Case Western for the

---

[32]Letter from K. S. Warren to G. R. Pomerat, Associate Director Medical and Natural Sciences, The Rockefeller Foundation New York. 10 August 1965. **The RF archive.**

[33]Andrade, Z.A. and Warren, K.S. Mild prolonged schistosomiasis in mice: alterations in host response with time and the development of portal fibrosis. Trans. R. Trop. Med. Hyg. 58: 53–57, 1964.

Warren, K.S. Experimental pulmonary schistosomiasis. Trans. R. Soc. Trop. Med. Hyg. 58: 228–233, 1964.

Warren, K.S., Reboucas, G. and Baptista, A.G. Ammonia metabolism and hepatic coma in hepatosplenic schistosomiasis. Patients studied before and after portacaval shunt. Ann. Int. Med. 62: 1113–1133, 1965.

Warren, K.S. and Weisberger, A. S. The suppression of schistosomiasis in snails by chloramphenicol. Nature 209: 422–423, 1966.

past two and a half years and apparently has made quite an impact … Warren acted rather nervous, particularly during the early part of my visit, and at times his report of the studies which had been carried out in his laboratory was confused. The reprints which he will forward to us may clarify some of this. In any event some of his studies have included the following: (1) a study of the penetration of the cercariae of S. *mansoni* in common laboratory animals. The cercariae will penetrate the skin of mice, hamsters, rabbits, and guinea pigs, but maturation of the cercariae occurs mainly in mice and hamsters. The presence of water is required for pene-tration. Warren has also found that the cercariae penetrate dead animal skin as readily as living tissue. Having been intrigued by this, he also found that cercariae penetrate lima beans. On the basis of this he has obtained a number of specimens of tropical plants, and of about 20 varieties studied, he has found one, the butterfly lily, which seems to attract cercariae and which is actively penetrated by them. This particular lily came from the Philippines and Warren does not know its distribution in tropical areas but this observation presents the possibility of control methods. (2) Warren has become interested in agents which inhibit protein synthesis. The Head of the Department of Medicine, Dr. Austin S. Weisberger, reported an observation at the recent Federation meetings in Atlantic City concerning the role of chloramphenicol as an inhibitor of protein synthesis in cells. Working with Weisberger, Warren has found that chloramphenicol in high dilution prevents the development of schistosomes in snails."[34] The early anxiety that Scott noted was not detrimental; the precision of Warren's experiments and his clarity of thought and dedication were to secure him a patron and passage to St. Lucia.

Prioritising his work over family life, the young Ken Warren gradually expanded his research interests, raising his scientific profile and helping him to attract talented researchers to the laboratory.[35] One of the first people to have a career-defining position at the Institute of Pathology was the Filipino, Dr, Ernesto "Ernie" Domingo. Writing and working shoulder-to-shoulder with Warren, he learned to prosper within the demanding and uncompromising regime that infused the labo-ratory. Both men were interested in granuloma production in experimental schis-tosomiasis and attempted to determine whether this was related to immunity and/or hypersensitivity. Because granuloma production can be inhibited in animals treated with immune-suppressive agents, Domingo studied the effects of thymectomy and X-irradiation. Ernie worked in Cleveland for only a few years, but it was a period during which he refined his scientific thinking, published prolifically—including 12 scientific papers within the space of 2 years—and identified the clinical subjects

---

[34]Excerpt from the diary of V. C. Scott, Visit to Case Western Reserve University Cleveland, 24 May 1966. The **RF archive.**
[35]K. S. Warren & J. H. Dingle, "A study of illness in a group of Cleveland families. XXII. Antibodies to *Toxoplasma gondii* in 40 families observed for ten years." N. Engl. J. Med. 274: 933–997, 1966.

that would be his lifework.[36] Warren's autocratic, peremptory management style certainly forced a high tempo and high productivity: The joke in the laboratory was, "He wants tomorrow's data for yesterday."[37] An aggressive researcher with an insatiable appetite for data, ideas, and new areas of research, Warren similarly displayed an easy dexterity working across disciplines while attracting good collaborators interested in fibrosis, anemia, immunity, and immunology. Later in his career, Domingo won the prestigious Ramon Magsaysay Award for his work in the Philippines where he organised and led the Liver Study Group until 2001. The group did major work on viral hepatitis including hepatitis A, B, C, D, E, and G, and this work—together with his investigations of *Schistosomiasis japonica*—prevented millions of premature deaths in the region.

Another scientist whose career trajectory was defined by Warren was Dov Boros, the RF-sponsored Israeli immunochemist. Boros spent 6 years in Cleveland, and there Warren's influence was decisive on his future by introducing him to immunoparasitology. On 17 June 1968, Warren travelled to the RF offices in New York to meet Virgil C. Scott. Free from nerves, his true emotions came to the fore: "KSW came in bubbling over with enthusiasm about his schistosomiasis research. Working with Boros, who has been with him less than a month, they have found that the material in the egg responsible for the development of the hypersensitivity state related to granuloma formation is soluble in the supernatant fraction of centrifugal eggs destroyed in ultrasonification."[38] One of the most profound scientific influences on this new work had been the 1966 publication, "Delayed hypersensitivity," by the distinguished New York based immunologist, J. W. Uhr.[39] This publication captivated Warren and he immediately began to apply its philosophical underpinning to research, thus leading him to apply irradiation and chemotherapy to the schistosome egg. However, it was with Boros and their joint publication in 1972 that further experimental advances were made with a ground-breaking study that isolated soluble egg antigens from parasite eggs. These antigens, when injected into experimental animals, induced a delayed-type hypersensitivity, later renamed "T-helper lymphocyte–mediated immune response."[40] The major breakthrough established that the glaucomatous cellular reactions that appeared around the deposited eggs were immune responses to the egg antigens, not to the egg-induced

---

[36]K. S. Warren & E. O. Domingo, "Granuloma formation around *S. mansoni, Schistosoma haematobium* and *japonicum* eggs in unsensitsed and sensitsed mice: Size and rate of development, cellular composition, cross-sensitivity and rate of egg destruction." Am. J. Trop. Med. Hyg. 19: 292–304, 1970; K. S. Warren, M. S. Rosenthal & E. O. Domingo, "Mouse hepatitis virus (MHV3) infection in chronic murine schistosomiasis mansoni." Bull. N. Y. Acad. Med. 45: 211-224, 1969.

[37]Dov Boros, personal communication.

[38]Excerpt from the diary of V. C. Scott. 17 June 1968. The **RF archive.**

[39]J. W. Uhr, "Delayed hypersensitivity#2". *Physiol Rev.* 46 (3): 359–419, 1966.

[40]D. L. Boros & K. S. Warren, "Delayed hypersensitivity-type granuloma formation and dermal reaction induced and elicited by a soluble factor isolated from *S. mansoni eggs*." J. Exp. Med. 132: 488–507, 1970.

irritation as previously believed. This discovery helped to elevate the profile of Warren, his co-workers, and Case Western Reserve University to the scientific community in the US and beyond.

Boros and Warren had good interactions, often walking together from the laboratory toward their homes in Cleveland Heights. This civilised co-existence was tested during the write-up of their collective work, which took 2 years before Warren and Ms Taylor (the fearless departmental secretary, lector, and final arbiter of style and content), would allow the paper to go to press. Although Boros brought new skills to the laboratory, Warren's persistent push for new data resulted in daily tensions as acknowledged by Boros: "I've had my frustrations and triumphs while working in his lab. We had an interesting dynamic; he was the mentor, but I had the needed expertise in the rapidly evolving delayed hypersensitivity, later cell-mediated immunity field. Ken had a keen sense in how to apply those newly emerging immune parameters to the pathology of *S. mansoni*, and our publications in the murine model influenced the field of clinical schistosomiasis."[41] Boros became a celebrated immunoschistosomologist at Wayne State University, (Detroit, Michigan), and he still thinks about Ken Warren with "fond gratitude" for getting him started in immunoparasitology.[42]

S. mansoni was a chronic granulomatous disease that affected approximately 200 million people in the tropics, and Warren soon wanted to expand his knowledge of the disease outside the controlled environment of the laboratory. To this end, he constantly lobbied Virgil C. Scott to financially support a research project on St. Lucia. Scott eventually acceded, and as a first step it was agreed that a 4-day fact-finding visit should take place in June 1968. Ostensibly this was to evaluate how Warren's ideas would combine with the RF's ongoing research projects, but of equal importance was to assess the personality dynamics of the forcefully enthusiastic Warren and the Englishman, Peter "Pip" Jordan, the director of RF's field station. After the initial visit to the field station, Warren, in a lengthy phone call to Scott, put his benefactor's mind at rest. The entry in Scott's RF diary reads: "KSW reports on his St. Lucia visit. Initially, he found PJ 'a little hostile since he didn't know why I was there' but the atmosphere gradually warmed up over a few beers and all ended up amicably, he feels. The question of schistosomiasis infection vs. disease was discussed at length. On the basis of PJ's figures on hepatosplenomegaly and after seeing eight or ten affected patients, KSW feels that there is a lot more disease than PJ and Lees have been aware of. KSW feels that the only way to answer the question as to the cause of this syndrome in St. Lucia is combined liver punch biopsy and spleno-portagraphy in a dozen selected patients. KSW is willing to collaborate in this and feels it may be possible to carry out these procedures in St. Lucia … In short, KSW feels there are a number of problems that need study that he

[41]Dov Boros, personal communication.

[42]D. L. Boros & K. S. Warren, "Effect of antimacrophage serum on hypersensitivity (*S. mansoni egg*) and foreign body (divinyl-benzine copolymer bead) granulomas." J. Immunol. 107: 534–539, 1971.

and others at Case Western Reserve can be helpful with, and he is anxious to formalise a relationship … For a five-year project he estimates he would need approximately $12,500/year or a total of $65,000 … I would be willing to consider initial support at the grant-in-aid level. KWS is a real fireball and I believe he could inject a lot of vigor into the programme."[43]

Two years later, with the funding in place, Warren, together with his family, went on a 3-month research visit to the RF's schistosomiasis field station on the island of St. Lucia in the Caribbean. The station had been established in 1965 with a memorandum of understanding signed between the government of St. Lucia and the RF. Each side "agreed to cooperate in the study of matters affecting the health of the people of St. Lucia and in seeking and applying measures to control disease and, more specifically, schistosomiasis."[44] The idea was to identify three valleys where the incidence of schistosomiasis was high and, during a period of years, system-atically apply one of the three known control methods. Then the effects, benefits, advantages, disadvantages, and the costs would be assessed.

The person who had been chosen to direct this audacious undertaking was Dr. Peter "Pip" Jordan, a veteran of the tropics. He had previously performed a trial of filariasis control on an island in Lake Victoria, Tanzania, but was prevented by the government from expanding the study; thus his research interest had shifted to schistosomiasis. A brilliant researcher trained at the London School of Hygiene and Tropical Medicine, Pip Jordan typified the image of the colonial doctor that Patrick Manson might well have encountered in the Victorian era. Strong, large of build and charismatic of nature, sleeves rolled-up, ready for action, he wore the uniform of the earlier Colonial Medical Service: white shorts and knee-length white socks with the tops turned down with impeccable tidiness.[45] Some might have suspected that on meeting Jordan, Warren would have seen him as anachronistic; after all, he believed that "tropical medicine" was a pejorative term, irrevocably linked to the colonial era, and that it was not merely moribund but dead and buried. But far from it, on a personal level, after their first awkward meeting, the men got on well, collaborating on many research projects on St. Lucia. Both enjoyed drinking single malt whisky while talking science in the evening, and most surprisingly of all, Warren also embraced the traditional colonial uniform of white shorts and knee-length white socks!

Jordan recruited another American, Joe Cook, to his staff to oversee the clinical management of patients presenting with schistosomiasis, and during the 1970s Warren, Cook, and Jordan collectively made enormous contributions to the study of

---

[43]Excerpt from the diary of V. C. Scott. 12 July 1968. The **RF archive.**

[44]J. Goodfield, *Quest for Killers,* Companion volume to the PBS Television Series: Hill and Wang, 1987, p. 107.

[45]J. Goodfield, *Quest for Killers,* Companion volume to the PBS Television Series: Hill and Wang, 1987, p. 109.

morbidity and immunity in human *Schistosomiasis mansoni*.[46] Prominent among these advances were a series of papers on passive transfer of immunity.[47] Moreover, Warren's and his colleagues' studies on the immunology of schistosomiasis were performed in China, Egypt, the Philippines, and St. Lucia, which established features of immunopathology and components of resistance (Fig. 1.1).

Life on St. Lucia was heavenly for Sylvia Warren and their children, Christopher and Erica, who stayed in the Malabar Hotel for three consecutive summers playing on the beach with Joe Cook's three small daughters and other children who found themselves on the southern end of the Caribbean for scientific reasons. Ken Warren was happy, too; his new status allowed him the opportunity to use the RF's field station to persuade scientists to study the intractable characteristics of schistosomiasis. Among with this group was the Harvard immunologist, John David, who was "seduced" by Warren "to explore the tangled fields of immunoparasitology."[48] At an immunology meeting in 1972, Warren, knowing that David was working on transfer factor, talked to his colleague about his own work with granulomas in the Caribbean and his desire to conduct an experiment to see what transfer factor could do given that men who worked in the drainage ditches, who because they had very high delayed sensitivity to schistosomiasis, didn't seem to have the disease.[49] David then replied, "My wife, Roberta, and I have been working on transfer factor." "Really," Warren countered, "fantastic! Would you be willing to come to St. Lucia to do this?" "What is St. Lucia?" the immunologist answered![50]

Warren got his way. John David, his wife Roberta, and their two children spent the summer of 1972 on St. Lucia—paid for by Warren—working with Joe Cook and Pip Jordan to investigate whether transfer factor had any role in schistosomiasis.[51] This experiment was an outlier for Warren's later Great Neglected Diseases Programme, which aimed to attract highly motivated and skilled scientists into parasitology. The quest soon showed innovative outcomes: John and Roberta David made the very first ever lymphocyte proliferation with schistosomiasis while on

[46]J. A. Cook, S. T. Baker, K. S. Warren & P. Jordan, "A controlled study of morbidity of schistosomiasis mansoni in St. Lucian children, based on quantitative egg excretion." Am. J. Trop. Med. Hyg. 23: 625–633, 1974; K. S. Warren, J. A. Cook & P. Jordan, "Passive transfer of immunity in human schistosomiasis mansoni: Effects of hyperimmune antischistosome gamma globulin on early established infections." Trans. R. Soc. Trop. Med. Hyg. 66: 65–74, 1972.

[47]Cook JA, Warren KS, Jordan P: Passive transfer of immunity in human schistosomiasis mansoni: Effect of transfer factor on early established infection. Trans Roy Soc Trop Med Hyg. 69: 488–493, 1975.

[48]K. S. Warren & C. C. Jimenez (eds), *The Great Neglected Diseases of Mankind Biomedical Research Network: 1978–1988*. New York: The Rockefeller Foundation, 1988, p. 15.

[49]Transfer factors were originally described as immune molecules that are derived from blood or spleen cells that cause antigen-specific cell-mediated immunity, primarily delayed hypersensitivity and the production of lymphokines, as well as binding to the antigen themselves.

[50]John David, personal communication.

[51]K. S. Warren, J. A. Cook, J. R. David & P. Jordan, "Passive transfer factor of immunity in human schistosomiasis mansoni: Effect of transfer factor on early established infections." Trans. R. Soc. Med. Hyg. 69: 488–493, 1975.

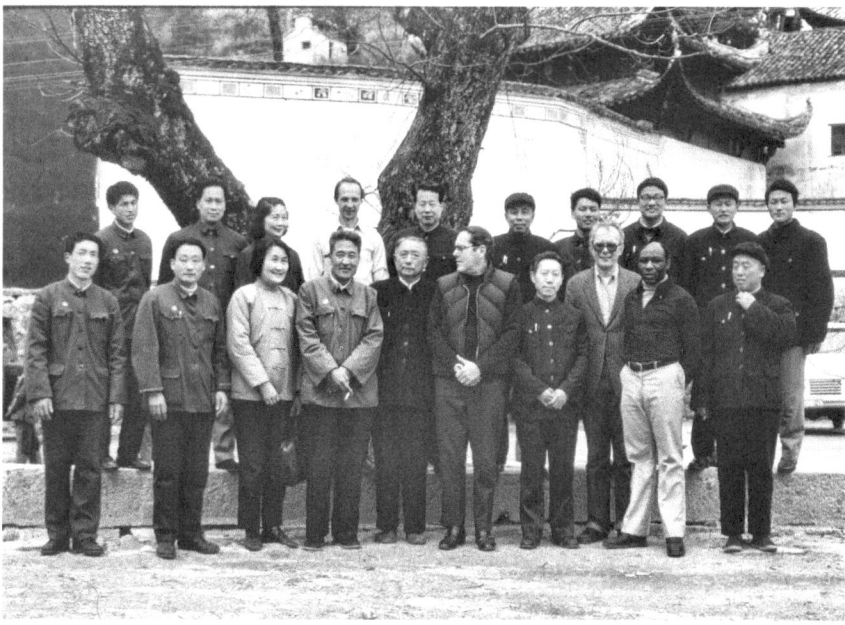

Fig. 1.1 *Left* to *right, top row*, Joe Cook (4th). *Left* to *right, bottom row*, Chinese political 'minder' (1st), Professor Su, (5th) with whom Ken had arranged the study of mortality in schistosomiasis japonica in rural China. Ken Warren (6th), Ken Mott (8th), then head of schisto for WHO, Pierre Peters (9th), a technician for many years at Case-Western Reserve (who worked with Warren, Adel Mahmoud, and Charles King). Courtesy of Christopher Warren. A paper resulted from this study—Warren, K.S., Su Delong, Xu Zhao-yue, Yuan Hong-chang, Peters, P.A., Cook, J.A., Mott, K.E., and Houser, H.B. Mortality in schistosomiasis japonica in relation to intensity of infection. Study of two rural brigades in Anhui Province, China. N. Engl. J. Med. 309: 1533–1539, 1983

St. Lucia. This was not their only novel brainchild: Needing some carbon dioxide (CO_2) for an experiment, but with none on the island, they asked their teenage daughter, Lisa, who was due to join them for the summer vacation, to collect a tank from their laboratory in Harvard and bring it to St. Lucia on the plane. It is difficult to imagine such a request in today's more fearful world, but Lisa duly did what was asked of her and flew to the Caribbean with the tank of CO_2 on her lap! John David later became an integral part of the GND programme, becoming the first director of the renowned Biology of Parasitism Course at the Marine Biological Laboratories in Woods Hole, Massachusetts, which transformed the teaching of the subject in the USA.

In autumn 1970, after his first visit to St. Lucia, Warren spent a year as visiting professor at the London School of Hygiene and Tropical Medicine. Back in London, Warren, the "terrific Anglophile," felt liberated.[52] He rented a small home

---

[52]Adel Mahmoud, personal communication.

in Dulwich for Sylvia and the children, and soon, Christopher excelled at Dulwich College, whereas Erica, a smart and vibrant 5-year-old, enchanted her classmates at the James Allen Girls School with stories of tarantulas on St. Lucia. Sylvia, too, was elated to be back in London, geographically close to her family, and she felt culturally and psychologically at home, unencumbered by American strictures and mores. At the LSHTM, Warren's students were exposed to his zest for life; he encouraged them to enjoy the thrill of science, to embrace a willingness to be wrong, and to admit that they didn't necessarily have all the answers. The overwhelming impression was one of enthusiasm, and this was catalytic, changing the trajectories of scientific careers with a combination of charm, loyalty, and unbendable determination.

The year at LSHTM would also be a decisive episode in Warren's life because there he met Adel Mahmoud, who became his close friend, most important scientific collaborator, and protégé. Mahmoud, born in 1941, studied at the Cairo Medical School before completing a doctorate programme at the LSHTM, and he shared a common interest in schistosomiasis with Warren. Originally from Egypt, where the disease was endemic, Mahmoud had wonderful stories about his experiences working at a rural health unit after he had finished medical school. Over the years, Adel became an "adopted son" of the Warrens', and the year in London was punctuated by visits to London restaurants, introduced to them by Patrick Hamilton, a young assistant professor at the LSHTM. Warren loved to eat, and many happy evenings were spent in a Greek restaurant in Bayswater and the Swiss Centre at Leicester Square. A close personal bond quickly established, and 2 years later when Mahmoud, again over dinner in London, voiced his wishes to join Warren's laboratory as a post doc, Sylvia looked at him solemnly and said in disbelief, "Do you really want to leave London for Cleveland?" "No," came the reply, "but the science is important."[53]

A year later, Mahmoud was at Case Western and was immediately catapulted into Warren's swirling centrifugal work ethic: hypothesis, experiment, publish; hypothesis, experiment, publish … Warren's infectious speed and focus led to the publication of their first scientific paper together only 10 weeks after Mahmoud had arrived in Cleveland.[54] Mahmoud recognises that his career in medicine took a more illustrious path when he decided to join Warren in Cleveland: "If I had stayed in London, which would have been very attractive, I would have been a carbon copy of the old professors in England. If I had gone back to Egypt, I would have been a dead loss. So this was a phenomenally important step."[55] Mahmoud and Warren established a very productive scientific relationship and worked together in Kenya, the Philippines, Egypt, and China. In 1974, in Kenya, Warren, together with Mahmoud and his team, performed a pioneering programme of "selected population

---

[53]Adel Mahmoud, personal communication.

[54]A. A. F. Mahmoud, K. S. Warren & D. L. Boros, "Production of a rabbit anti-mouse eosinophil serum with no cross-reactivity to neutrophils." J. Exp. Med. 137: 1526–1531, 1973.

[55]Adel Mahmoud, personal communication.

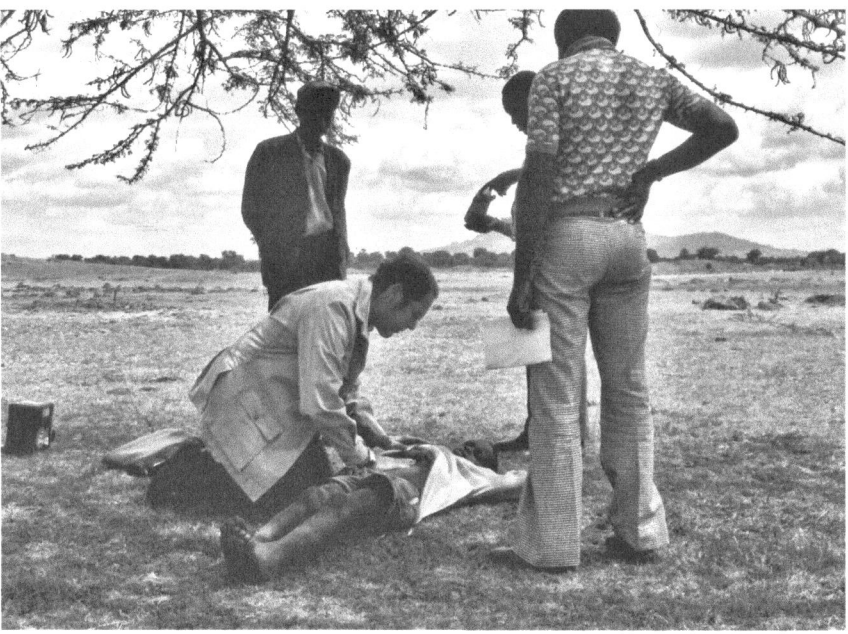

Fig. 1.2 Ken Warren examining a child in the Machakos district, Kenya, 1974. Courtesy of Christopher Warren

chemotherapy," a term he himself had coined. Under this scheme, urine and stool samples from an entire population were examined, but only the people excreting schistosome eggs—mainly children and young adults—were treated with the hope that treatment would not need to be repeated many times: a policy that the WHO now adopts today. The Case Western Reserve years witnessed the high-water mark of Warren's scientific career: In less than two decades, he stood at the forefront of American tropical medical research. The extent of his achievement, galvanising and energising the science and practice of the subspecialty, was highlighted in Mahmoud's 1996 obituary of his friend and colleague: "Our fundamental current concepts of the cell-mediated basis for granuloma formation, its down-regulatory mechanism, and its central role in pathogenesis of schistosomiasis are but a few of Ken's multiple contributions… His most influential contributions relate to a modern understanding of the epidemiology of infection and disease in populations of endemic areas, which led to the current universal approach to control using targeted chemotherapy (Figs. 1.2, 1.3, and 1.4)."[56]

---

[56]Adel Mahmoud, obituary of Kenneth S. Warren Journal of the American Medical Association, February 5th, 1997. Vol. 277, No 5, p 429.

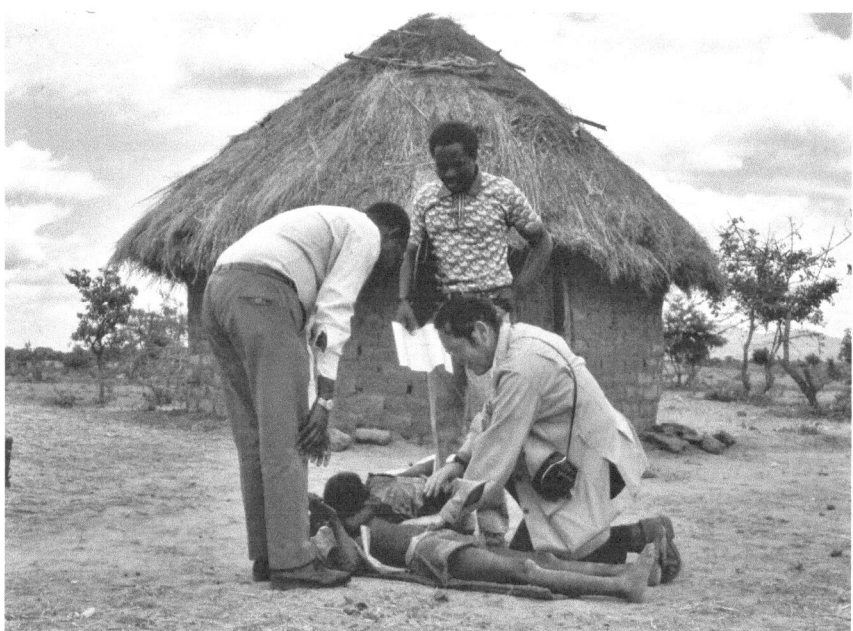

Fig. 1.3 From the bench to the bush, Ken Warren working in the field, Machakos district, Kenya, 1974. Courtesy of Christopher Warren

Recognition of Warren's dedication to tropical diseases came in an equally inimitable manner: In 1974, he was appointed Director of the newly established Division of Geographic Medicine at the Case Western Reserve Department of Medicine. This was the first such institution in academic American medicine devoted to diseases in the developing world. This was a liberating appointment in a number of ways: It moved Warren out of the Institute of Pathology, which had been John Dingle's small fiefdom; furnished him with a unique new position funded by a $525,000 grant from the Rockefeller Foundation; and allowed him to focus exclusively on infectious diseases and the secondary illnesses arising from them ranging from malnutrition to cancer. A central task of the division was to target helminthic and diarrheal diseases, which were a major cause of paediatric illness in the US. A combination of the strong base in clinical medicine at Case Western Reserve, together with the high-quality research output of Warren and his colleagues, was decisive in persuading the RF to establish the new institution in Cleveland. Ideas had been forming in Warren's mind for some time about the nature, direction, and wider relevance of physicians interested in the health problems of developing countries. As he noted, "geographic medicine has too long been separated from the mainstream of medicine. It has been carried on in this country by

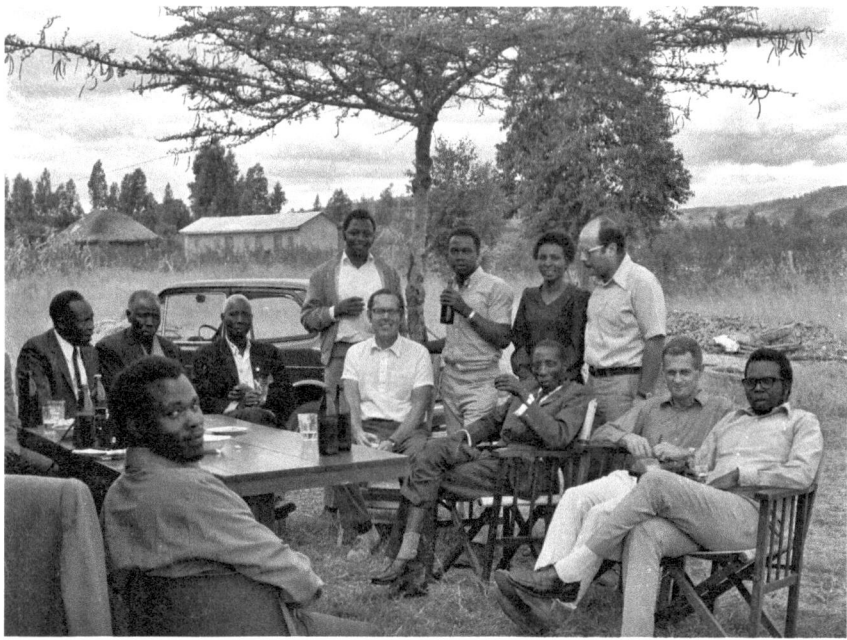

Fig. 1.4 This photograph records the first meeting of Warren with the chief of the Kamba tribe, John Ouma. Courtesy of Christopher Warren

public health schools and government agencies, and in Europe by specialised schools of tropical medicine."[57] Instead, Warren sought to reintegrate his discipline back into the wider modern biomedical field (Fig. 1.5).

Warren was extremely fortunate in having Dr, Charles "Chuck" Carpenter, Professor and Chairman of the Department of Medicine, as an enthusiastic ally. Carpenter had made many contributions to the treatment of cholera while he was director of the Johns Hopkins Centre for Medical Research and Training in Calcutta from 1962 to 1964, and he strongly supported the programme and its ideals. Unified by the alchemy of experience and prescience, both men believed that a career avenue now existed for physicians interested in health problems of the developing world. These major diseases affected 80% of the world's population, and advances in the understanding and management of many epidemic and endemic diseases of developing countries would have world-wide impact as well as provide significant feedback to medicine in general. Chuck Carpenter arrived at Case Western in 1972, and was immediately impressed by the precision of Warren's research and his enthusiasm. He recalls, "Ken did a lot to show how life-expectancy varies much

---

[57]Medlines to Case Western Reserve School of Medicine, January 1974, p. 1.

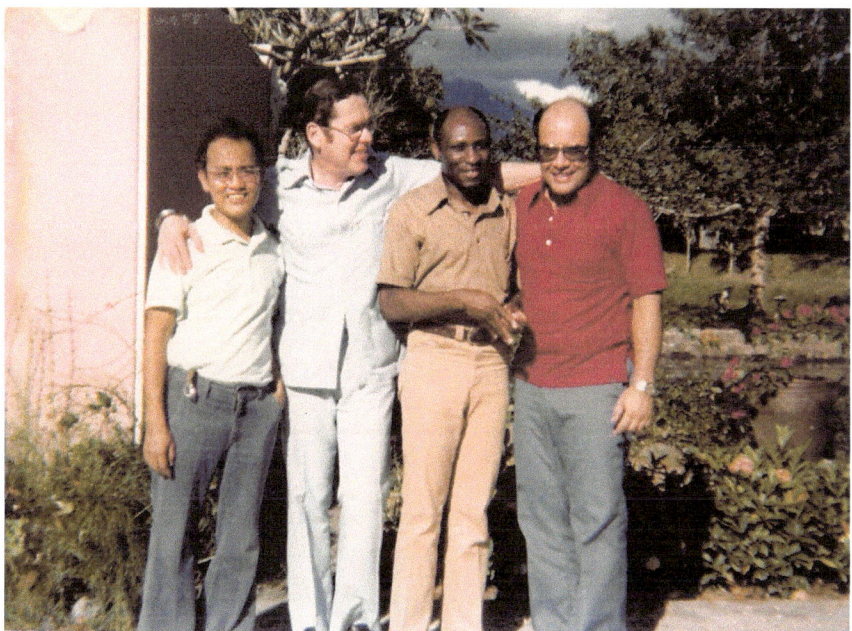

Fig. 1.5 Ernesto 'Ernie' Domingo, Ken, Pierre Peter, and Adel Mahmoud. Courtesy of Christopher Warren

throughout the world. He brought that to people's attention. Also, tropical medicine in the US was a lack-lustre specialty and I gave him money rather than to the cardiologists."[58]

The upward parabola of Warren's career continued in 1975 when he was awarded the prestigious Squibb Award of the Infectious Diseases Society of America. The accolade was presented annually to a medical investigator for outstanding accomplishment in the field of infectious diseases, and its award signified to the wider world that Warren was now an authority in tropical medicine—he had arrived. More garlands came his way, among them memberships of the National Library of Medicine, the editorial board of Experimental Parasitology, the American Association of Immunologists, the Edna McConnell Clark Foundation, and the Council of the American Society of Tropical Medicine and Hygiene. As an ambitious investigator with a love and aptitude for writing, Warren's proudest honour was inclusion in the Institute of Scientific Information: 1000 Contemporary Scientists Most Cited, 1965–1978. Warren did not, however, limit himself to his burgeoning career in the laboratory. Unusually for any academic, he crossed traditional disciplinary boundaries by combining his love of medicine with a keen interest in library science, a field in which he also held a professorship at Case

---

[58]Charles Carpenter, personal communication.

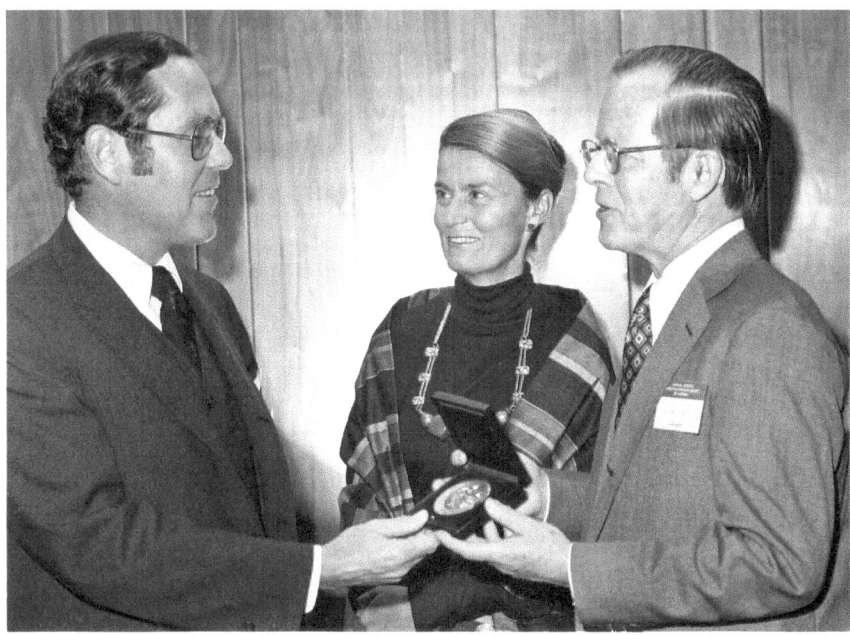

Fig. 1.6 Thomas Huckle Weller presenting Ken with The Squibb Award of the Infectious Diseases Society of America, 1975. Sylvia looks on with a sense of pride and amusement. Courtesy of Sylvia Warren

Western Reserve. This was a rare confluence of two distinct disciplines, which had been cross-fertilised by his friendship with William Goffman, another Professor of Library Sciences at the university. For both men, scientific communication in the 1970s was in a disorderly state, and they set out to enhance the quality of communication by applying a mathematical model and bibliometrics, which was defined as the statistical analysis of published literature.[59] Warren's fascination with schistosomiasis, communication theory, and information systems led him to write two major scholarly bibliographic works chronicling the entire literary history of the disease over a 100-year time period (Fig. 1.6).[60]

It was undeniable to all that knew him that Ken Warren excelled at self-promotion. But he was also very welcoming, an excellent host, possessed an infectious personality, and always willing to promote his colleagues and collaborators. Christmas and Thanksgiving celebrations at the family home at 2917 East

[59]K. S. Warren & W. Goffman, "The ecology of the medical literatures." Am J. Med. Sci. 263: 267–273, 1972.
[60]K. S. Warren, *Schistosomiasis: The Evolution of a Medical Literature. Selected Abstracts and Citations, 1852–1972.* The MIT Press, Boston, 1973; K. S. Warren & V. A. Newill, *Schistosomiasis: A Bibliography of the World's Literature from 1852 to 1962.* 2 vols, The Press of Western Reserve University, Cleveland, 1967.

Overlook Road were always liberally sprinkled with members of the Case Western Reserve family. Moreover, he made a point of taking Boros, Mahmoud, or Domingo to conferences to introduce them to influential figures and to generally use his media savvy skills to promote his colleagues. NBC news even ran a curious piece on Warren's laboratory that juxtaposed the internecine war involving Egypt and Israel in 1973 and the harmony and peaceful co-existence between those countries' nationals at Case Western Reserve![61]

Warren's scientific influence at Case Western grew as he continued to champion the global burden of schistosomiasis on the world's poorest people. He believed that the disease could be prevented and treated when the mechanisms responsible for it were clearly understood, and all of his ingenuity and inventiveness were directed toward this mission. This endeavor had brought him professional fulfillment and scientific success but little financial reward. Although Warren was an MD and had served as an intern at Boston City Hospital, he had not done his mandatory 2 years of residency and had rejected clinical medicine in favour of the laboratory. In a period of self-reflection, he lamented "the rigors of an under-paid academic career with no advanced clinical training and no income whatsoever from patients…," realising that his salary was always going to leave him an impecunious relative to his high-rolling cardiologist colleagues.[62] As a consequence he was restless, and had seriously pursued job opportunities at the London and Liverpool Schools of Hygiene and Tropical Medicine and the Bernhard Nocht Institute for Tropical Medicine in Hamburg, Germany. This was not the only cost incurred by his life scientific: If Warren possessed an "intense scientific ambition," so too Sylvia wanted to excel in her chosen field. After all, when they had met in London, she was independent, career-minded, and well educated—in essence a modern day feminist. Marriage brought a more conventional lifestyle, and whereas Sylvia enjoyed motherhood and had a profound nurturing influence on Christopher and Erica, she had to forgo the earlier professional period of her life. Although it was true that she found time to redesign the British Club in Bahia and worked part-time as an interior decorator in Cleveland, the demands of Ken relocating the family across the world meant that this sphere of her life effectively atrophied. The compensating creative force in her life was gardening; for the rest of her life Sylvia cultivated beautiful gardens that are a living testament to her hard-work, artistic design, and invention. Their garden at 2917 East Overlook Road was one of the finest in Cleveland Heights, and although strapped financially, Sylvia maintained an elegant home and was a renowned host and legendary cook (Figs. 1.7 and 1.8).

One inescapable feature of Warren's life, discernible early in his career, was his polarising personality. Having worked with Warren for 24 years, John David was well placed to reflect on his colleague's "two characters." Although readily acknowledging that, "outside of my family, nobody changed my life as much as

---

[61]Dov Boros, personal communication.

[62]K. S. Warren, Speech given on 19 June 1996, Picower Institute for Medical Research. Courtesy of Sylvia Warren.

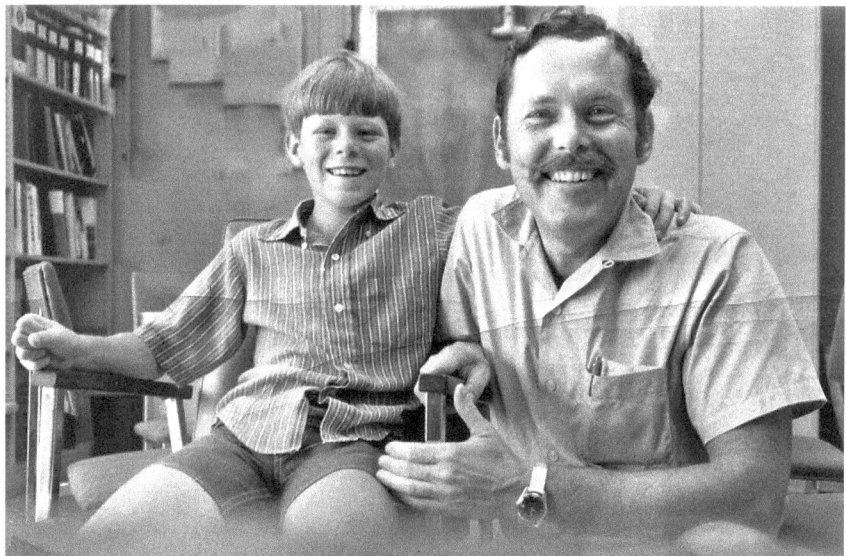

Fig. 1.7 Ken and his son, Christopher. Courtesy of Christopher Warren

Ken. There is no question, going into parasitology, starting the Woods Hole course, ending up being Chairman of the Department of Public Health at Harvard, all of that would never have happened without Ken Warren," and being dazzled by Warren's vision, brilliance, loyalty, and commitment to helping the poor of the world, David noted that these qualities were tempered by his friend's tendency to "go overboard about what *he* did, what *his* people did, and other people didn't count."[63] For Warren's benefactors and beneficiaries, this created a warm glow, but for those outside his circle it fermented ambivalence and resentment. His polarising personality would prove a stumbling block, and David evaluated it in unambiguous terms: "He was his own worst enemy." Such tensions were obvious in an encounter with Tom Weller, with whom Warren had past history. Weller, a virologist, was Head of Tropical Public Health at the Harvard School of Public Health, and his influential status in the field was strengthened in 1954 when he was awarded the Nobel Prize in Physiology or Medicine for his research on polio. Warren looked on Weller as insufferable and conceited. At a meeting of the American Society of Tropical Medicine, Warren exceeded his allotted presentation time by a few minutes, and was immediately informed by Weller, the session chair, "Your time is up Ken, please leave or stop." But Warren refused, and finally, he almost had to be removed bodily from the stage. It was an unpleasant episode, and Weller never forgot or forgave Warren.[64] It is probably no coincidence that Weller was never

---

[63]John David, personal communication.

[64]Dov Boros, personal communication.

Fig. 1.8 Ken and his daughter, Erica. Courtesy of Erica Warren

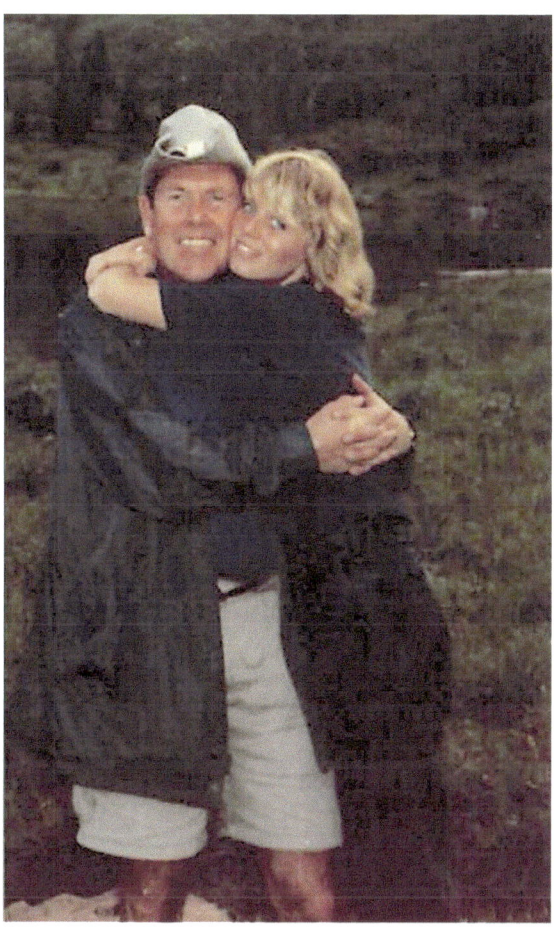

invited to Cleveland until Warren left in 1977, and Adel Mahmoud became the Chair of Medicine. It was clear to all that Warren was a dynamic investigator who enjoyed the thrill of science. He could see what needed to be done, and he would pursue it single-mindedly; that was his talent. But at the same time he could offend people, and although they may not have become enemies, these were people who theoretically could, if they so wished, support him. Events, such as that with Weller, were amassing and working against him (Fig. 1.9).

Despite his sometimes abrasive personality, Warren continued to break new ground. His passion to bring the new biological sciences to infectious diseases was reflected in the "Mechanisms of Disease" course he designed and taught at Case Western. Meanwhile, the scientific salesmanship and energy he deployed so successfully in pushing—and sometimes overstating—the debilitating burden of

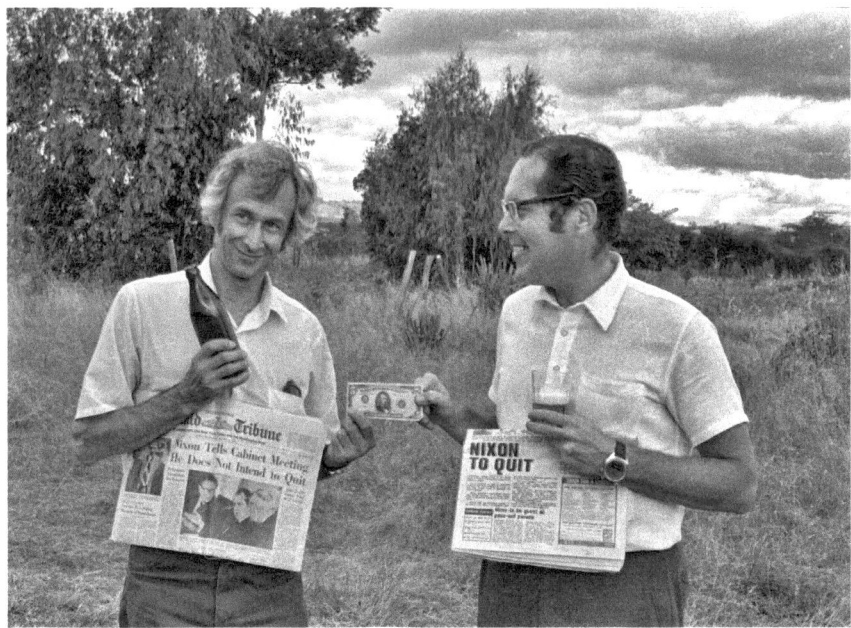

Fig. 1.9 Following the Watergate scandal and subsequent cover up, Richard Nixon resigned the presidency on August 9th, 1974. Even though John David was holding the NY Times which said that Nixon would not resign, John won the $5. Courtesy of John David

schistosomiasis earned him a reputation as being a man of ideas and action. He had shown himself to be a trusted custodian of the RF's first-ever Division of Geographic Medicine, which required the careful disbursement of a large grant, and the running of a programme that had important implications for physicians interested in health programmes in developing countries. This increased level of exposure and responsibility suited Warren's personality; his zest for life, enthusiasm, ambition, and dedication to biomedical science were now paying off. However, in a fateful concourse of atoms in the void, illness was to temporarily disrupt the tangent of progress. A tumor was discovered under Warren's arm, and he immediately underwent surgery at Case Western. On investigation, the initial diagnosis was that the tumor was benign and that the prognosis was good. However, a short time later, nodes were discovered, again under his arm, and when the slide from the original operation was re-examined, the tissue was found to be cancerous. The cancer was identified as malignant melanoma, and a series of further operations followed, including a splenectomy, resulting in a large number of nodes being removed from his body. Warren was in his mid-forties, Erica was 12, and Christopher was 17, but far from capitulating or complaining, Warren faced his disease with the same attitude as he had lived his life, i.e., with an attitude that anything was possible. At the beginning of 1977, his medical colleagues reassured

him that all of the metastatic lymph nodes had been removed, and he was pronounced cured.

More ambrosia followed. Warren was invited by John Knowles, President of the
RF, to come to New York and discuss the possibility of joining him on an ambitious
mission to promote the well-being of mankind throughout the world. The two men
could not have been better suited. Knowles was a swashbuckling figure. The first
physician to be president of the RF, with a distinguished medical career, he was
highly regarded for his enthusiasm, intellect, and good humour. As a student at
Harvard, he had made extra money as a left-handed jazz pianist in a speakeasy in
Scollay Square, Boston. Similarly to Warren, Knowles was a dynamic man, famous
for campaigning for health reform in the US, but he had a particular set of problems
at the RF where he had inherited a stagnant health programme. He felt constricted
by life-long employees, "lifers" as he referred to them, who prevented rather than
promoted new ideas. With their imminent retirement, and with the injection of
Warren's vision and vigour, Knowles saw an opportunity was at hand to take the
RF to the next stage. The previous 5 years of his presidency had focused primarily
on the problems of population, size of the family, and ways of achieving population
stabilisation, all of which related to the health of the family and the community.
Internally at the RF, there was also some policy friction between Knowles and the
retired Chairman, John D. Rockefeller III, but Knowles was determined to finally
get hold of the Health Division and allow Warren the opportunity to spearhead new
advances in the basic sciences related to the great neglected diseases.[65]

For his part, Warren had already formulated in his mind a synthesised programme, which would include targeting diarrheal and respiratory diseases, malaria,
schistosomiasis, African sleeping sickness, hookworm, and other infectious diseases. This was the very programme that Knowles had envisaged bringing him to
the RF to do. However, before Warren could accept the post of Director of Health
Sciences, he felt compelled to tell Knowles about his recent illness. Knowles was
unperturbed, commended Warren for his honesty, and said, "No, you're the man I
want."[66] Paradoxically, within 2 years, Knowles would die from pancreatic cancer
at the age of 52. He died leaving a wife, six children, and a truncated legacy at the
RF; it would fall to Ken Warren to see their collective dreams fulfilled. Of course,
with Knowles's death, Warren had lost his great defender, supporter, and collaborator. His wish to supercharge parasitology in particular and tropical medicine in
general would now be embarked on without his formidably able and protective
colleague. On a personal level, Knowles's death was a warning, and Warren began
a programme of immunostimulatory BCG injections to activate lymphocytes with
the hope that they would prevent any future recurrence of the melanoma. He
recognised what might be coming: He had a lot of work to do and a finite time in
which to do it.

---

[65]Lincoln Chen, personal communication.
[66]Sylvia Warren, personal communication.

Chapter 2
The GND Years

Warren was an immediate beneficiary of the changing philanthropic principles that Knowles began to introduce at the RF and, with his customary drive, he immersed himself in the opportunities that arose from this redefined strategy. One of Knowles' first acts was to add the title of Health to the foundation's Population Programme, which subsequently became known as Population and Health. Previously, under the presidency of the biologist George Harrar, health programmes, with the notable exception of the St. Lucia schistosomiasis research, had grown peripheral to the core concerns of the foundation, which were oriented toward agricultural development.[1] The Conquest of Hunger Programme of the Agricultural Sciences Division fostered the so-called "Green Revolution" for which one of its officers, Norman Borlaug, received the Nobel Peace Prize in 1970. When Warren arrived at the RF in July 1977, annual expenditures in the area of health, other than those related directly to the Population Programme, were less than 2% of the foundation's disbursements. The appointment of Warren, a tropical medicine specialist, marked a watershed departure from recent policy; however, at the same time, it adhered to the traditional interests of the RF. After all, its philanthropic genealogy can be traced to the success of the Rockefeller Sanitary Commission in 1913 and the inauguration of a major global hookworm control campaign. Key international public health activities followed in the 1930s and 1940s when the foundation played a significant part in the control of malaria and yellow fever, for which a foundation officer—Max Theiler—received the Nobel Prize in 1950 for developing the yellow-fever vaccine.[2]

Knowles had hired Warren for a specific purpose—to focus on the debilitating infectious diseases of the forgotten three quarters of the world's people in devel-

---

[1]The Conquest of Hunger Programme of the Agricultural Sciences Division fostered the so-called "Green Revolution," for which one of its officers, Norman Borlaug, received the Nobel Peace Prize in 1970. The prize was awarded to Borlaug for his pivotal role in helping modernise agriculture in the developing world, an effort known as the "Green Revolution." The phrase was first used in 1968 by William S. Gaud, former director of United States Aid for International Development (USAID).

[2]J. P. Kreuer (ed.), *Malaria, Immunology and Immunization*, Academic Press, 1980, p. 336.

© Springer International Publishing AG 2017
C. Keating, *Kenneth Warren and the Great Neglected Diseases of Mankind Programme*, Springer Biographies,
DOI 10.1007/978-3-319-50147-5_2

oping countries. It was a concrete problem, and Warren set himself the objective of finding the most cost-effective form of medical intervention to help reduce the sequence of "exposure, disability, and death."[3] Warren adopted a numerical view of global health and was firm in his belief that the lives of children in poor countries mattered just as much as those of children in richer geographies. Everyone scored the same in terms of the metrics of importance with the aim to achieve good health care at low cost. Through his constant exposure to and interaction with other medical scientists, Warren became greatly interested in diarrheal and respiratory diseases (the biggest killers of children), neonatal death, and the delivery of vaccines. His great project, which was a unique idea at the time, was to combine known excellent active groups already working on tropical medicine, with an emphasis on tropical diseases, especially parasites, with other scientists in the nascent fields of immunology and molecular biology. Although this latter group may have had no previous experience in tropical disease research, Warren recognised the achievements of the founding fathers of the discipline of parasitology and had indeed been inspired by them to enter the field. However, scientific medicine after World War II had greatly accelerated as a result of the increased professionalisation of research. Of course, fine work was still being performed in parasitology, but for Warren the discipline had somehow remained immune to the infusions of excitement, experimental advance, and forward momentum that were occurring in biology. Revolutionary developments were happening in molecular and cell biology, but parasitology was not transformed in the same way as virology had been for example. Furthermore, the experts who had a profound understanding of specific tropical diseases lived and worked in countries where the infrastructure for first-class research was poor or non-existent. As the celebrated Australian research biologist, Gus Nossal, who first met Warren in 1976, noted, "It is no disrespect to many fine parasitologists to say that, in the third quarter of the twentieth century, their discipline slipped behind the times." Now with the financial backing of the RF, Warren's vision was to apply this "new biology" to parasitic diseases, particularly malaria and schistosomiasis, in the developing world. It would not be too much to say that Warren wanted to change the world's structure.[4]

The Rockefeller years marked the high-water point of Warren's career. In the 1960s and 1970s, the RF had been in the business of growing crops, slowing population growth, and providing public-health initiatives around the world while at the same time consciously attempting to avoid becoming entangled in the internal politics of beneficiary countries.[5] This philosophical position became a point of internecine contention that underscored the profound differences within the RF about the value and the role of Western science in the developing world. Warren entered the debate wholeheartedly on the side of those who continued to advocate

---

[3]J. A. Walsh & K. S. Warren, "Selective Primary Health Care: An Interim Strategy for Disease Control in Developing Countries," N. Engl. J. Med. 301: 967–74, 1979.

[4]Gustav Nossal, personal communication.

[5]Kenneth Prewitt, personal communication.

for the role of Western science in ameliorating the social problems of developing countries. Although some contended that this view bore all the marks of hubris and that true salvation should come through the alleviation of poverty, which was the true root of the burden of disease, Warren believed there was no time to waste in waiting for such conditions to come about. As such, the RF offered him, in his own words, a "truly unique" opportunity to fulfill his visions. He had great freedom within the organisation, and providing he could read the prevailing policy mood, he could build on the great American tradition of scientific philanthropy by coupling science and scholarship to foster the RF's noble ambition to promote the "good of mankind throughout the world," Indeed, Warren's belief in science formed a historical precedent with the legendary RF officer Warren Weaver, who for a generation had been the architect of programmes in the natural sciences.[6] Weaver had been brought into the foundation in the early 1930s to apply the ideas and methods of the physical sciences in biology. Weaver, like Warren, was a taxonomist and is credited with the first use of the term "molecular biology." He too eschewed peer review in favour of his own personal selection of grantees, just as Warren would do.

Inside the offices of the RF on the Avenue of the Americas in New York, the atmosphere was conducive, as it had been in the 1920s, to the idea that the foundation's primary purpose was to facilitate the programmes of its directors. These directors played a pivotal role in the working of the organisation, acting as a bridge between the foundation's trustees and field programmes. Experts in their own specialties, these officers, including Warren and the head of Agricultural Sciences, Norman Borlaug, were autonomous and trusted custodians of their divisions, well respected in their fields, and accountable only to the RF board. On occasion, members of the board were well-informed individuals, e.g., when Theodore "Ted" Hesburg, President of Notre Dame, was chairman of the RF. However, in general, they were not experts on parasitic diseases or geographic medicine, and there was little in the way of peer-review adjudication of new internally conceived research projects. This did not mean that programmes in Warren's Health Sciences Division were not the end result of rigorous debate and intellectual examination. John Knowles wanted what he called "scholar activists" on his staff: people who had deep knowledge of their programme's subject matter, who were respected for their own research and scholarship, and who had a vision of how this research and scholarship might be applied to solve social problems worldwide. Warren unreservedly embraced this ideal, feeling it was incumbent upon him to remain active to the best of his ability in his field of scholarship, to keep up to date with the literature, and indeed to continue to contribute to this body of knowledge.

In August 1978, the philosopher John Bruer was interviewed for the post of Visiting Research Fellow and became the first person to be hired by Warren as Director of the Health Sciences Division. "At the interview Ken said that he *needed* a philosopher. He believed in the ideals of scholarship and he encouraged others to follow his example, which I think was admirable of him and the RF at that time.

---

[6]*The Rockefeller Foundation 1913–1988*. RF publication, p. 12.

Also, Ken brought his knowledge and vision to one of the most important positions in international philanthropy and health. He taught us to make a good programme, the importance of finding the best advisors and grantees, and how to build an intellectual and institutional infrastructure to support new research areas. As a grant-maker, Ken was both entrepreneurial and enthusiastic—two rare traits."[7]

Warren may have believed that he "needed" a philosopher for three specific purposes. First, he valued the humanities and saw the benefit of recruiting a non-scientist scholar into his circle. Another primary reason was Warren's awareness of the ethical issues surrounding health and population work in the developing world. Third, a more tangential reason lay in his interest in information and information systems. Bruer had previously worked in quantum mechanics and had some abilities in lattice and graph theory. Graph theory has provided the analytical background for much work in bibliometrics as well as complex systems research. In 1988, Warren and his colleague, William Goffman, published a bibliometric analysis of the papers published by the Great Neglected Diseases of Mankind Programme.

This commitment to science owed much to the contemporary self-confidence of the scientific community and the growing sense that science and medicine increasingly had the capabilities to mediate all kinds of previously intractable social ills, an ambitious and optimistic mindset exemplified by the publication of the Yarborough report in 1970 that advanced a strategy for the "means and measures necessary to facilitate success in the treatment, cure and elimination of cancer—at the earliest possible date."[8] Warren embraced the 'can-do' attitude, and placed himself in the slipstream of the feel-good factor that was deeply entrenched at the RF in the 1970s. The foundation was still riding the wave of its Green Revolution, and its enormous historical accomplishments, so why couldn't the future be an intimation of the past? Why couldn't there be a breakthrough in male contraception, in vaccine discovery, and in the mechanisms of parasitic diseases?

Genesis and Recruitment

Warren was faced with a scientific and administrative challenge—how to attract outstanding scientists in the burgeoning fields of molecular biology, immunology, and biochemistry to work on the great neglected diseases in the developing world. He began by sketching the outline of a new programme that would target such illnesses by harnessing and funding the collective talent of leading scientists from around the world.

In December 1977, Warren presented his proposal to the Board of Trustees of the RF. The document suggested how the great neglected diseases of mankind could be addressed by the creation of "a network of high-quality investigators who would constitute a critical mass in the field, attract the brightest students and

---

[7]John Bruer, personal communication.

[8]National Programme for the Conquest of Cancer, *Report of the National Panel of consultants on the Conquest of Cancer,* US Government Printing Office, 1970.

conduct research of excellence."[9] The great neglected diseases were described as "great" in terms of prevalence and "neglected" because they affected neglected people. Warren wanted to remodel the historic ideals of the foundation to couple philanthropy and basic science to help address the disproportionate inequity of the global poor. In particular, the synthesised programme would target diarrheal and respiratory diseases, malaria, schistosomiasis, African sleeping sickness, hookworm, and many other infectious diseases. An essential component was the establishment of research units in the mainstream of modern biomedical investigation housed within universities, medical schools, and great scientific institutions. Importantly, the programme affirmed one of Warrens' sacrosanct ideals, that "a significant part of the investigator's efforts would be spent in applied collaborative research with colleagues in developing countries."[10] In this sense the project would establish global networks linking "the bench to the bush."[11]

The idea of attracting numerous groups of carefully selected researchers in both developed and developing countries to focus on parasitic diseases was both innovative and controversial. Focusing on "neglected" diseases certainly proved provocative. For some, the word was suggestive of the fact that errors had been made in how and where financial and intellectual capital had previously been channelled.[12] Yet Warren was unapologetic in attempting to reorient and reinvigorate the field. Although outstanding work had been performed in descriptive parasitology earlier in the century, by the 1970s the discipline had failed to adopt the revolutionary changes that had been taking place in molecular and cell biology, genetics, and immunology. By emphasizing the collaborative and interdisciplinary fusion of research from around the globe, Warren's GND network was poised to revolutionise the ways in which infectious tropical diseases were investigated by representing the first attempt to apply modern biomedical technology in the elucidation of mechanisms of disease prevalent in developing countries and bringing research on the latter to the mainstream of medicine in developed countries. The project was also a departure from tradition in terms of how it would be funded. As a researcher himself, Warren knew only too well the frustrations of writing grant applications, the trepidation of not having a grant renewed, and the general administrative obstacles to actually getting on with the work. To avoid these strictures and to smooth the progress of research, he advocated that all of the GND grants would be guaranteed for a period of 8 years, an unusually long period of time that gave researchers financial security and freedom.

---

[9]K. S. Warren & C. C. Jimenez (eds), *The Great Neglected Diseases of Mankind Biomedical Research Network: 1978–1988*. New York: The Rockefeller Foundation, 1988, p. 1.

[10]K. S. Warren & C. C. Jimenez (eds), *The Great Neglected Diseases of Mankind Biomedical Research Network: 1978–1988*. New York: The Rockefeller Foundation, 1988, p. 1.

[11]G. F. Mitchell, in K. S. Warren & C. C. Jimenez (eds), *The Great Neglected Diseases of Mankind Biomedical Research Network: 1978–1988*. New York: The Rockefeller Foundation, 1988, p. 49.

[12]Hans Wigzell, personal communication.

Warren successfully sold the idea to the RF board by emphasising the foundation's long history in international health and that the time was now ripe for new ground to be broken. The formal tenets of the new undertaking were as follows:

- Research would range from the basic level in highly sophisticated laboratories through clinical investigation and field epidemiology and anthropology.
- Research would be investigator-initiated in terms of the problems approached, which could be any aspect of any of the "great neglected diseases."
- Support would be for at least 8 years and would be flexible, although emphasis would be on the development of young investigators and on international collaborative research.
- The units would be gathered into a global network for communication and collaboration fostered by annual meetings. Fourteen foundational units were to be recruited and established with the only mandatory requirement being that high-quality collaborative science was undertaken and that members would attend annual meetings of the GND.

Thus, the Great Neglected Diseases of Mankind Network was born. With the concept and research objectives in place, Warren spent the best part of a year persuading some of the world's leading scientists to bring their chosen specialties into tropical medicine. In addition to persuading several American colleagues to join the GND, he established collaborations with scientists across the world in Egypt, Israel, Australia, Thailand, Sweden, England, and Mexico. It was a truly interdisciplinary group bound together by Warren's ability to persuade good scientists to work on diseases in which he was interested and, in some cases, in which they had shown scant curiosity. He achieved this with a combination of bonhomie, enthusiasm, and the mutual respect of those working with him.[13] Of course, there was no peer-review committee and no consensus; the entire group was selected single-handedly by Warren.

The impetus to get the project off the ground relied almost entirely on Warren's strength of character and his personal evolution as a scientist. For Warren, four distinct elements were necessary: (1) to tempt some of the best minds in medical science into the field of tropical medicine; (2) to apply the most sophisticated methods and ideas to the work; (3) to expose these teams recruited from outside traditional tropical medicine to the realities of the diseases in the field; and (4) to create intellectual and personal connections between the different teams, to fuse them into a strike force whereby the whole was greater than the sum of its parts. To achieve this, Warren used his inherent strengths as a catalyser, proselytiser, and matchmaker. He prided himself on his personal network, on knowing *everyone*.

Key to the recruitment process was to convince outstanding individuals who were not currently working in tropical medicine that they should consider a change of direction. This Warren did with consummate ease. Antony Cerami, the world-renowned biomedical scientist, was at Rockefeller University in 1977 and

---

[13]Keith McAdam, personal communication.

looks on his first meeting with Warren as career defining: "The first time I met Ken was a memorable and unique experience. Over lunch, Ken painted in broad strokes but very bright colours, this vision of what was to be subsequently known as the GND. The dedication of Ken to the field of parasitology and the poor people of the world is an aspect of the GND that I will never forget. He managed to instill these thoughts in everyone. It was the most important lunch of my life, since it launched me into new unknowns with a group of dedicated people that I am proud to be associated with."[14] Many of the enlisted "high-class investigators" echoed this sentiment and recognised that the GND had a profound influence on their careers and personal values.

To advise the network on immunology, Warren courted a giant of translational immunology, the President of Israel's Weizmann Institute, and President of the International Union of Immunology, Michael Sela. Perhaps it was their shared Jewishness—although Warren didn't wear his Jewishness on his sleeve and was highly secularised—or their internationalism, or a commitment to using science to alleviate suffering, but there was an immediate empathetic understanding between the men. Sela found Warren to be an "infinite charmer" and they became close friends almost immediately. Sela believed that the idea of the GND was "terrific" and that the people selected "were not only good scientists, nice people, but also had the quality to collaborate together... which was all part of the success." Sela admired Warren's ideas, the zeal he brought to the project, and he particularly valued another trait of Warren's from which he benefited personally: "Ken was what is called in Yiddish a 'shadkhen', a matchmaker, and matchmaking is very important. I met Shelley [Sheldon] Wolff through Ken and he became a great friend. When I finished my ten years as head of the Weizmann, I moved to Tufts in Boston, where Shelley was Chairman of the Department of Medicine. Shelley was very important: he was a leader, and while I was an advisor on immunology, Shelley performed the same role for infectious diseases [as part of the GND network]."[15]

One of the outstanding physicians already on Wolff's staff at Tufts was Gerald "Jerry" Keusch, who went on to become director of the Fogarty International Centre for Global Health at the NIH. Jerry had finished his training in infectious disease in 1970 and hoped to pursue a career in what is known today as "global health." After spending some time in Bangkok trying to understand the mechanisms of cholera, he later became interested in the relationship between malnutrition and the susceptibility of children to recurrent infection. By the time he was recruited to Tufts in 1978, he was a pioneering physician in the nascent field of molecular medicine. At the time, there was no formal relationship between the RF and Tufts, and so Wolff set up an appointment for Jerry to meet Warren in the hopes that they might join the network and secure much-needed funding. In many respects, Keusch fulfilled the criteria that Warren was looking for: He had experience of working in the field; he

---

[14]Anthony Cerami, personal communication.
[15]Michael Sela, personal communication.

would be mentored by his friend Shelley Wolff; and he fully intended to make his career studying infectious diseases in developing countries. Still, there was a lot riding on the meeting, and Jerry felt a sense of trepidation when he learned that their get-together would take place at the Infectious Diseases Society Conference in New York, in October 1978: "We met, and he sits me down in the middle of a staircase, where everybody is going up and down. Kind of a classic Ken move; he's conducting an interview and people are walking by, everybody who wanted one of the RF grants was stopping and tapping him on the shoulder in a 'remember me?' way. Anyway, I guess I passed [the interview] because we got the award and took the job in January 1979."[16]

In a similar fashion, Warren also persuaded Hans Wigzell to join the group. Wigzell at the time was working on the immunology of murine malaria at Uppsala University in Sweden. Just how unorthodox the GND programme was seen to be was evident from the men's first meeting. Warren travelled to the Karolinska Institute in Stockholm where Wigzell introduced him to the institute's president, Sune Bergstrom, himself a Nobel laureate. Wigzell remembers Bergstrom's bafflement at the GND concept as he asked his colleague, "This strange American, what is he actually doing? It's strange...?!" Bergstrom was unable to visualise how the new programme would work in the context of traditional research methods.[17]

Warren was also keen to recruit a specialist in molecular medicine and quickly convinced the Oxford-based physician–scientist David Weatherall (at the time working on inherited disorders of haemoglobin in the tropics) and his team to join the network. Indeed, the new link would prove fortuitous for Oxford medicine in general because the university's leading reputation in international health for developing long-term north–south research partnerships and capacity building in tropical medicine can be traced to a seemingly innocuous meeting between Weatherall and Warren on a dark misty evening in 1977. The two men met in London, and as Weatherall admits, "when Ken first told me about the GND programme over an excellent dinner at a slightly decadent hotel near Victoria, I was quite sceptical. [But] in the words of the poet Oliver Goldsmith, 'fools who came to scoff remained to pray.' When he told me that the Rockefeller would offer research support for a minimum of eight years and that the only stipulation was that we met annually with the other groups to exchange information, I decided to go ahead."[18]

With the majority of the key players selected, Warren's Great Neglected Diseases project began operation. The network would eventually span five continents and placed Warren at the forefront of tropical medical research. Each unit was deliberately situated within existing departments of medicine so as not to be divorced from clinical skills and clinical understanding in terms of pathogenesis and mechanisms of disease—essentially the science of identifying vaccine

---

[16]Gerald Keusch, personal communication.

[17]Hans Wigzell, personal communication.

[18]David Weatherall, personal communication.

candidates, drug targets, and diagnostics. Initial components of the GND included divisions of geographic or tropical medicine at Case Western Reserve University, Tufts University, the University of Virginia, the University of Washington, Oxford University, and the Biomedical Research Centre for Infectious Diseases in Cairo, Egypt. Immunology units were established at Harvard University, the Walter and Eliza Hall Institute in Australia, the universities of Stockholm and Uppsala in Sweden, and the Weizmann Institute, whereas pharmacology units were in action at Rockefeller University, Case Western Reserve University, the Centro de Investigacion y de Estudios Azanzados in Mexico City, and Mahidol University in Bangkok, Thailand. All of the groups were to spend approximately 30% of their time in collaborative research in the developed world with countries such as Kenya, Egypt, Sudan, India, Guatemala, Brazil, Malaysia, Gambia, Indonesia, and Papua New Guinea. The investigators worked mainly on bacterial diarrheas and helminth and protozoan infections.[19]

The Network in Action

The first meeting of the GND was held at the Abby Aldrich Rockefeller Hall, New York, in 1978. It was an unforgettable experience. Warren had invited two giants of British parasitology, George Nelson and Philip Marsden, to the event to elaborate on the new possibilities of applying modern specialties to the old field of parasitology. The two men were great raconteurs, full of mind-expanding stories gathered over decades working in the tropics and thrilled the group by signposting the ways in which the new biomolecular sciences might affect old diseases. Marsden was a legendary figure in tropical medicine with research interests in insect-borne protozoal disease. He worked in both Africa and South America and was a professor of medicine at the University of Basilia for 17 years. In Gambia, West Africa, he performed one of the first longitudinal studies of tropical child health, which led to his doctoral thesis. One event that occurred while he was a medical officer in Gambia colourfully describes his idiosyncratic and highly adaptive remedial style: "While water surfing in the Atlantic the Governor trapped a large Physalia jellyfish between his chest and the surf-board. I was fishing off the beach at Mile 5 and they brought him to see me. The red wheals were already visible on his chest from the discharged nematocysts on the tentacles. Fortunately I had a full bladder, so immediately I urinated on his chest to wash off the residual nematocysts and had people throw sand on his chest while I ran to the car to get some morphia. After much pain he made an uneventful recovery."[20] Meanwhile, George Nelson was one of the world's most distinguished parasitologists; a former medical officer in Uganda and researcher at the division of insect-borne diseases in Nairobi, he ended his academic career in parasitology at the Liverpool School of Tropical Medicine. The friendship,

---

[19]Warren described parasitology as, "a biological discipline concerned largely with two separate groups of organisms—single-celled protozoa and the multi cellular metazoan of which the helminths form the most important group".

[20]*A Jubilee Scrapbook 1947–1997. An anthology of tales and photographs depicting 50 years of the MRC in The Gambia. Collected by* A. Greenwood, J. Foster, H. Pickering and M. Weber, p. 10.

camaraderie, and sense of fun that existed between Warren and Nelson are borne out in an exchange of letters between the two men:

> Dear George, What a pleasure to receive your enthusiastic letter about 'a marvelous safari' in the Sudan and Kenya. Sylvia and I had the great pleasure last March of going up to Lake Turkana by land, an incomparable experience. I also had another incomparable experience and that was developing chronic diarrhea which I brought to China with me and back before I realised that it was our old friend the Giardia…[21]

For the uninitiated, Nelson and Marsden gave a perspective that none of the GND team possessed because they had spent decades in the tropics coping with parasitic assault. Moreover, at the time, British parasitology was far ahead of the discipline anywhere else in the world, and in addition to being full of inspiring stories, Nelson and Marsden knew the field's literature intimately. Keith McAdam attended the meeting at the Abby Aldrich Hall as part of Shelly Wolff's team from Tufts: "Marsden and Nelson were two eccentric champions of tropical medicine. They taught a week's course on parasitology which was quite something for a group of biomedical scientists who were into the new age of immunology and molecular biology. They just thrilled us with all the possible involvement of new skills in developing answers to the diseases they described."[22]

With only three or four scientists from each of the units present, the meeting was characterised by its intimacy and held in an atmosphere that oscillated between excitement, optimism, apprehension, and relaxed creativity. It marked the fulfillment of an audacious ambition: to bring new bio-molecular scientists to the field of parasitology, to create intellectual and personal connections between the different units, to stimulate competition as well as collaboration, and, ultimately, to improve the human condition. In a wider context, the subsequent flowering of invention within the GND was partially attributable to the breadth of intellectual perspective that informed the scientific work during the period. The group represented an interdisciplinary ideal that was the very antithesis of the divided world described by C.P. Snow in 1959 as a 'society split into the two titular cultures—namely the sciences and the humanities'.[23] Warren prided himself on his undergraduate studies at Harvard and was eager to point out that it was not always necessary to have a first-class degree in biochemistry to be a physician. There were other backgrounds that would be helpful, and several of his GND colleagues had backgrounds in the liberal arts, which played perfectly into one of Warren's favorite aphorisms: "there are many rooms in the house of medicine."[24]

Each year the meetings became bigger and more rambunctious. Close friendships were established between many outstanding researchers, and the annual event became rather like a reunion or perhaps a family gathering. At one of the early

---

[21]Letter from K. S. Warren to G. S. Nelson, Department of Parasitology, Liverpool School of Tropical Medicine, Pembroke Place, Liverpool, England. March 17, 1987.

[22]Keith McAdam, personal communication.

[23]C. P. Snow, Rede Lecture, 7 May 1959.

[24]John Bruer, personal communication.

meetings in the US, David Weatherall's team was invited to give a series of papers. The Oxford team had built up a strong partnership with the thalassaemia group in Thailand, which was led by Prawase Wasi, who had a habit of giving his lectures squatting on the floor in Buddhist style. Weatherall wanted his colleague to emphasise in his talk the importance of the RF to their work, and "not in the least because of the financial implications, I asked Prawase if he would lay on the thanks very thickly at the end of the lecture. He did say that he had had some success with the control of thalassaemia in Thailand but now they had been blessed in their endeavors because God had brought them Ken Warren. My immediate reaction to this rather excessive praise was to try and put my head under the seat!"[25] Later meetings took place in locations as far afield as Woods Hole, Massachusetts, a game park in Kenya, a hotel in Tel Aviv, a ski resort in Canada, and an Oxford college but with the continuing unifying objective to report on the past year's work, progress, and developments, to share knowledge, ideas, and doubts, and to create a sense of common goals and joint destiny. As observed first-hand by Sylvia Warren, the atmosphere was conducive to a huge degree of productivity: "They got an enormous amount accomplished at their meetings, and then they got on with their work afterwards because there were no impediments; they had long-term funding, so they didn't need to waste time filling in grant applications. It allowed them to produce, and how! (Fig. 2.1)".[26]

Of course, there were occasions when things did not run smoothly. In 1979, the second meeting of the GND programme was held at The Queen's College, Oxford. David Weatherall hosted the meeting and had gone to great lengths to provide an exciting scientific programme for the delegates and to make their stay in the city memorable. However, after spending one night in the historic but Spartan under-graduate accommodation, Shelly Wolff, muttering disquiet about the far-distant bathroom, decamped to the refined comfort of the Randolph Hotel! Similar dis-satisfactions were expressed about the catering provision because the Gothic setting was accompanied by a diet rich in carbohydrate and which had changed little since the days of Henry VIII. After the second day, with nobody showing up for college meals, David Weatherall was forced to make an appeal to his colleagues' humanitarianism, entreating them to "come to breakfast in the morning," because "the chef has threatened to commit suicide if nobody shows up."[27]

Research was at the heart of the GND's workings. Warren's philosophy was to develop the science, line it up with the clinical problems, and move between the laboratory and the clinic—the clinic, in the case of the GND, being the developing world. This was translational medicine in a developing world setting: the long road back and forth between the bedside, the laboratory, and the community. The main focus of each GND unit continued to be an examination of the mechanisms of

---

[25]David Weatherall, personal communication.

[26]Sylvia Warren, personal communication.

[27]Gerald Keusch, personal communication.

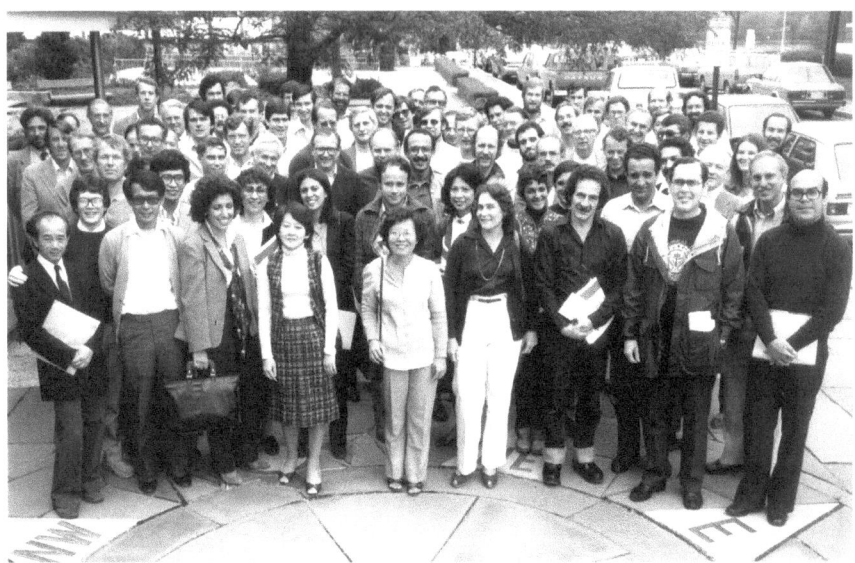

Fig. 2.1 Early 1980s meeting of the GND network at Woods Hole. Courtesy of Peter Hotez

disease, i.e., finding out how things worked. The innovative nature of the programme relates to a combination of applying genetic engineering technology to problems of parasitism; a belief that without fundamental investigations of the biology of these organisms as the major causes of disease, it would be very difficult to make progress in finding ways to control the disease. Importantly, the flexibility of the financial support allowed researchers to perform field work that would have been completely impossible under any other form of research grant. In this respect, the programme was prodigiously successful with groundbreaking work undertaken on the workings of numerous parasitic diseases including hookworm and schistosomiasis, although vaccines to such infections remain elusive even to this day. Rather, perhaps the most enduring legacy of the GND can be found in the transformations brought about in the financial modeling of such projects and the concomitant capacity to incubate new talent and collaborative work. The actuarial model of Warren's RF programme achieved remarkable results with only modest resources. During the 8-year period of its funded existence, the project involved 161 scientists and clinicians and 360 trainees, of which 150 were from the developing world, and resulted in the publication of 1800 papers. This was all accomplished at the cost of approximately $15 million ($55 million in 2015 values)—a prodigious rate of return on the investment by any standards.[28]

---

[28]K. S. Warren & C. C. Jimenez (eds), *The Great Neglected Diseases of Mankind Biomedical Research Network: 1978–1988.* New York: The Rockefeller Foundation, 1988, p. 2.

The funding policy of the RF transformed some of the units in the network from small laboratories working on model systems in mice into large bustling units with a stunning cadre of investigators who could attract additional resources. This was certainly the case at The Walter and Eliza Hall Institute of Medical Research, Melbourne, led by Graham Mitchell. Receiving GND funding enabled the Institute to expand its parasitology work by recruiting new researchers who would take part in the annual GND meetings alongside carrying out world-leading laboratory investigations. One such beneficiary was the immunochemist Emanuela Handman, who worked on leishmania. As a young, relatively inexperienced post-doctoral fellow at the time, Handman found inclusion into the GND network an "inspirational" experience that allowed her to rub shoulders with some of the greatest scientists of the era. She remembers these encounters as "open, friendly, and encouraging," while "the meetings opened new vistas of biology of which I knew nothing. This gave me the impetus and the confidence to move into new areas of research. As I moved on in my career, I started to realise how unusual the GND Network was. There was a sense of openness; the fact that junior or senior scientists did not hesitate to present the entire, uncensored data to all of the other participants. There was no sense of competition or secrecy; everything was on the table."[29] Being a recipient of GND support also meant that institutions were far more competitive when seeking other forms of external funding. Handman was the beneficiary of long-term funding from the NIH, WHO, and the Australian Society for Medical Research, all of which she acknowledges would "not have been possible were it not for the GND's seed funding. Moreover, the type of high-risk high-return work that we were undertaking would not have been fundable even for established parasitologists let alone newcomers Fig. 2.2".[30]

GND funding thus played a crucial role in expanding the horizons of parasitology by funding a talented group of young researchers who reinvigorated the status of tropical medicine in the United States and beyond. A brilliant cohort of scientists—including John David, Adel Mahmoud, Anthony Cerami, James Kazura, Gerald Keusch, Richard Guerrant, and Peter Hotez—were enticed by Warren to work on tropical diseases who otherwise might not have done so. In turn, all of these investigators have made a lasting contribution to disease control and human health, both as part of the GND programme and in subsequent years. Part of the reason why the network became such a formative experience in the lives of so many scientists was Warren's insistence that an important part of working in tropical medicine was to study in the field. This became a crucial component of the GND programme and in many cases a career-defining moment for those involved.[31]

---

[29]Emanuela Handman, personal communication.

[30]Emanuela Handman, personal communication.

[31]K. S. Warren, "The bench and the bush in tropical medicine," Am J. Trop. Med. Hyg. 30: 1149–1158, 1981.

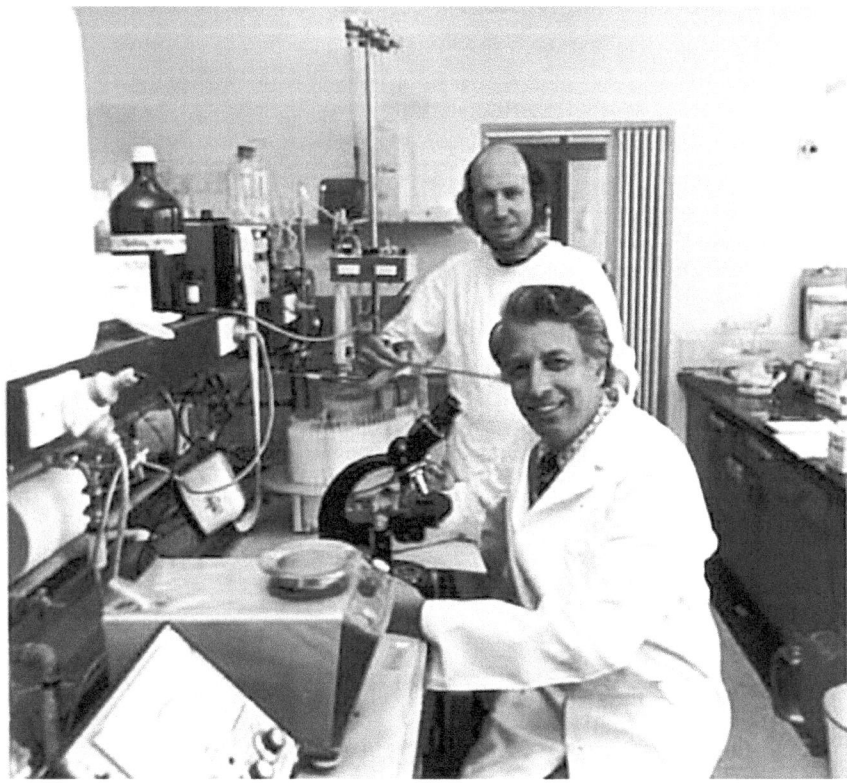

Fig. 2.2 Graham Mitchell and his boss, Gus Nossal (sitting), in the lab in Melbourne, Australia. Courtesy of The Walter and Eliza Hall Institute of Medical Research

Warren's own contribution to the story of schistosomiasis had revealed the crucial interplay between the "bench and the bush,"[32] and as the network developed and expanded, he encouraged his scientists to productively combine knowledge of the developing world with the powerful new tools of the "bench" into an effective synthesis. The benefits of this approach were clearly demonstrated by Anthony Cerami's experiences in the GND. Cerami ran his own laboratory in medical biochemistry at Rockefeller University, and through one of his MD/PhD students,

---

[32]In the tropics, clinical studies in hospitals and epidemiological studies in villages and among school children had shown the silent nature of the infection, even in patients with relatively advanced disease. The field investigation, which included the development of better parasitological methods for diagnosis, resulted in the collection of relatively large banks of parasitologically and clinically characterised sera. Meanwhile, work at the bench on the pathogenesis of schistosomiasis resulted in the development of an animal model, the characterisation of the parasite factor (egg) responsible for the disease, the essential role of the host inflammatory cell-mediated immunological response, and the occurrence of suppression of the host response by way of serum antibodies.

Steve Meshnick, he became interested in parasitic diseases in Africa. This led Cerami to spend time in Kenya observing the presence of cachexia in animals and people infected with parasites, work that marked the beginning of Cerami's search for the mechanism of this common occurrence of chronic disease, which is now known to be a macrophage protein produced in response to infection. On the back of this research, Cerami would later go on to co-write the patent that has become a landmark document in the history of anti-tumor necrosis factor (TNF) therapies.[33] Anti-TNF treatment of rheumatoid arthritis, Crohn's disease, and psoriasis has helped to improve the lives of millions of patients throughout the world.[34] Cerami's work was a vindication of Warren's concept of the scientific endeavour—Choose good people, fund them well, and let them rip!

Life in the field, however, did not always run smoothly. On one occasion, the native New Yorkers, Cerami and Meshnick, were taking in the local sites in Kenya. Unwisely, Steve thought that it would be a good idea to take his boss on a whirlwind safari at Nairobi National Park in his ancient Datsun. Within a short time they witnessed one of nature's most dramatic events: a lion killing and devouring its prey. The men got out of their car and cautiously took photographs of the scene. When they returned to the Datsun, however, it was stuck fast in the deep ruts in the road. Both men looked at each other and across at the blood-splattered lion. Cerami, the tenured professor, broke the silence: "Do you want to get out and push…?" Salvation came in the form of a Maasai tribesman, who, accustomed to the ways of the bush, walked across the open land, passed the salivating lion, and with the two laboratory-trained scientists looking on, perfunctorily eased the car out of the fissure to safety.[35]

Aberrations aside, Cerami readily acknowledges that the GND years were the most important in his life in science. His reflections capture the subtle equipoise between sacrifice and achievement that many biomedical scientists will recognise: "The annual meeting of the GND offered to each of us an opportunity to recharge our batteries to continue the hard, lonely work associated with science. The GND became a family dedicated to improving the well-being of mankind. The family aspects of belonging to a group had unique sociological effects. Every group wanted to show that they had established new and important scientific findings. Everyone wanted to look their best."[36] Perhaps most importantly, the meetings proved a focal point where researchers from geographically disparate parts of the globe could meet to collaborate across continents.[37] For young talented researchers at the beginning of their careers, it was exhilarating to talk, learn, and interact with

---

[33]A. Cerami, "A Surprising Journey in Translational Medicine," *Molecular Medicine* Vol. 20 (Supplement 1) 2014, p. s4.

[34]M. Feldmann, "Translating molecular insights in autoimmunity into effective therapy," Ann. Rev. Immunol. 27: 1–27, 2009.

[35]Steven Meshnick, personal communication.

[36]Anthony Cerami, personal communication.

[37]Keith McAdam, personal communication.

some of the world's brightest and most creative biomedical scientists including Michael Sela, David Weatherall, Gus Nossal, Peter Pearlman, and Shelley Wolff. This intellectual nexus brought professional recognition, that much needed antidote to the inevitable disheartening failures and loneliness of laboratory research. Acknowledgement and professional respect, experienced early in a scientific career, can have a life-long influence and strengthen resolve in difficult times.

Although the various units within the GND worked on very different aspects of parasites, from ecology, epidemiology, and immunology to infection and the genetics of host responses, the meetings offered an opportunity to foster new connections, particularly between researchers from the global north and south, as Warren had originally envisaged. An embodiment of the success of this ideal was the research on early childhood diarrhoea and enteric infections, undertaken by Dick Guerrant at the University of Virginia and Manasses Fonterles in Fortaleza, the capital of one of the poorest states in northeast Brazil. When Dick Guerrant attended the GND meeting in Oxford in 1979, he was 26 years old. He had trained as a paediatrician, just like his grandfather, and had begun his career in tropical medicine in the Congo before moving to Dhaka, Bangladesh, where the NIH ran a cholera programme. Working on cholera-stimulated oral-rehydration therapy (ORT), Guerrant sought to understand the mechanisms of secretory toxins to make ORT work more effectively, and it was this research that had brought him to Warren's attention. When Guerrant attended the meeting in Oxford, he invited along a stellar cast of colleagues: an expert on amoebic dysentery, Jonathan Ravdin; Ferid Murad, who would win the Nobel Prize in 1998; and the pharmacologist, Manasses Fonterles.[38]

For both Guerrant and Fonterles, the meeting marked the cementing of a working relationship, managed by Warren, that would endure for the next 35 years. Fonterles, a pharmacologist, possessed a good scientific genealogy, having worked with both Raymond Ahlquist and later with Julius Cohen in Rochester, New York, and had begun to work on the receptors that had important effects on the kidney and the gut. This research dove-tailed perfectly with Guerrant's own work on ORT, and so began the decades-long collaboration on enteric and diarrheal infections between the University of Virginia, the Makenzie Presbyterian University in Sao Paulo, and the village of Pakatuba in Fortelaza. This extended programme produced ground-breaking discoveries that would not have been made had it not been for the initial RF funding.[39] Guerrant is adamant that, far more important than any of his work on guanylate cyclase or adenylyl cyclase, was the discovery that high rates of chronic enteric and diarrheal infection lead to, on average, an 8-cm growth shortfall and a ten-point IQ deficit by the time children are 7–9 years old. With ORT, a child

---

[38]Ferid Murad shared the Nobel Prize in Physiology or Medicine in 1998 for showing that nitroglycerin and related drugs worked by releasing nitric oxide into the body, which relaxed muscles by elevating intracellular cyclic GMP.

[39]R. L. Guerrant, G. D. Fang, N. M. Thielman & M. C. Fonteles, "Role of platelet activation factor in the intestinal epithelial secretory and Chinese hamster ovary cell cytoskeletal responses to cholera toxin," Proc. Natl. Acad. Sci. Sept 27; 91 (20): 9655–9658, 1994.

will not die; mortality, although still high, has been decreasing, but morbidity is not. The collective work of Guerrant and Fonterles revealed the human and societal costs of diarrheal infection to the world's populations who continue to live in extreme poverty: It was a true translational partnership that successfully linked the laboratory to the clinic.

Warren, who retained a keen fascination with Brazil, having experienced his first true encounter with the "bush" there in Bahia in 1962–1963 while working on hepatosplenic *Schistosomiasis mansoni*, was the catalysing force that ensured the success and longevity of the partnership.[40] As a young researcher at the time, Guerrant admits to being "scared to death" at the beginning of the GND, but with Warren acting as a "masterful mentor," he was encouraged to follow his "wildest dreams."[41] Similarly for Manasses Fonterles, it was a chance encounter in Oxford with the colourful American who had opened his eyes to the possibility that his own scientific training could be used to help to identify the mechanisms of diarrheal disease in his native Brazil: "He made me believe that under his leadership a programme would not die and we started building bridges. He was a tremendous man, very energetic in defence of his ideas, in defence of the neglected diseases. At the time no one wanted to put money into them [neglected diseases] because the amount of return that you have will always be small … So for me, he was one of the most tremendous human beings that I ever met. The GND was the turning point in my life."[42]

A similar personal renaissance connected to Warren was experienced by Onesmo ole-MoiYoi, who grew up in a Maasai village in Kenya. His destiny as the community's cattle herder was irreversibly redirected by the power of education. More interested in books than being a trusted custodian of cattle roaming the edges of the Serengeti, Onesmo was sent by his father to school, where his dedication eventually won him an Aga Khan scholarship to Harvard. Reminiscent of Warren's own curriculum at the same university, Onesmo took a humanities degree before entering Harvard Medical School and specialising in immunology and molecular biology. Today, he is one of Africa's leading scientists and a forceful advocate for the application of more biomedical research to the continent's indigenous infectious diseases. Although Onesmo was never formally part of the GND network, he attended most of their meetings. Crucially, he had jettisoned the pathway of a conventional medical career for the study of infectious diseases after attending a lecture at Harvard in 1977 given by a proselytising Ken Warren: "Ken was talking about the idea of a network connecting leading institutions in the West with scientists in the developing countries, and in that lecture he mentioned the disproportionate amount of money spent on cardiovascular disease, diabetes and cancer, diseases considered important to the West, compared to the miniscule amount of

---

[40]K. S. Warren, "The bench and the bush in tropical medicine," Am. J. Trop. Med. Hyg. 30: 1149–1158, 1981.

[41]Richard Guerrant, personal communication.

[42]Manasses Fonterles, personal communication.

money spent on diseases of the developing world which affected millions of people."[43] At the time, ole-MoiYoi was working on the mechanism of hypertension, nothing to do with infectious disease, but the lecture, rather like his earlier disenchantment with herding cattle, brought unimagined change: "Meeting Ken was really a turning point in my life, because the numbers he gave showed that with minimal investment you could make a huge change in helping people to live healthier lives. Ultimately, a friend of Ken's, Barry Bloom, wrote a paper that mentioned a disease of livestock which transforms lymphocytes to become cancerous and kill the animal in three weeks. That caught my attention. Three years later, one of my professors, Donald Fawcett, went to Nairobi to set up an electron-microscopy laboratory in what is now called The International Laboratory for Research on Animal Diseases (ILRAD). A year later I went to Nairobi to work on the microbiology of this disease that transforms the lymphocytes to become cancerous. Meeting Ken, and listening to his lecture, was one of the things that led me to work on trypanosomiasis and malaria."[44] Indeed, the RF had a long-standing track record of supporting agriculture and animal care in the developing world. As early as 1943, CIMMYT, the International Maize and Wheat Improvement Centre, was established in collaboration with the Mexican Department of Agriculture to increase food crop production through research and development. Thirty years later, John Knowles was instrumental in providing the institutional framework for Onesmo ole-MoiYoi's career in East Africa by providing financial support for livestock research at ILRAD in Nairobi.

Warren and the GND

Warren remained very much at the epicentre of the network's activities, often by sheer force of his personality. Excitement, enthusiasm, and a sense of fun were the sentiments with which Warren infused his nascent recruits. His message was simple: Hubris and perfection are two of the enemies of getting things done, but enjoy the thrill of the science, and if you're lucky you will have some relevance to the people who suffer from infectious diseases. This he championed with great energy, and he found it difficult to take "no" for an answer. As one of his obituary notices observed, "this caused some to hide out until we were quite sure he was fully engaged in another project."[45]

Warren was certainly a "larger than life figure," an inherently charismatic and charming man, who in the words of Allen Cheever (who worked with him at the NIH in 1960), "was many things but never unenthusiastic and never modest. Ken saw what he wanted and got it."[46] He could also be bombastic, eccentric and swashbuckling, with a knack for "telling it the way it was … and sometimes

---

[43]Onesome ole-MoiYoi, personal communication.

[44]Onesome ole-MoiYoi, personal communication.

[45]R. Selzer, Kenneth S. Warren, M. D. June 11, 1929-September 11, 1996, *Molecular Medicine,* Vol. 2, No. 6, November 1996.

[46]John Cheever, personal communication.

rubbing people up the wrong way."[47] However, these perceived components of his personality were tempered by the recognition that he had a great vision for tropical medicine and the delivery of health services in the tropics. A more nuanced understanding of Warren's character is offered by his wife, Sylvia: "He did rub people up the wrong way, but somebody like that is bound to. Enthusiastic was probably the best way to describe him. Very focused, very sure of what he wanted to do, and very adept at finding the best way to do it."[48] John Bruer also recognised that Warren could be perceived as confrontational but that the loquaciousness, noise, and excitement could be open to misinterpretation: "He certainly didn't mind ruffling feathers, but I wonder if he even noticed that he was doing it … I don't think he set out to irritate people, I just think it was a function of his enthusiasm and drive. There was a single-mindedness to him, and that blinded him to problems and obstacles along the way. But Ken was always very kind personally, helping us younger people with our careers, and while he might get angry with Shelley Wolff or Ken Prewitt, he never got angry with us. There was that kindness that I think was at his core. He did some admirable things—you have to be in awe of the guy—but like all of us there were glaring deficiencies that got in his way."[49]

Warren was not helped in this department by the fact that the GND network's ethos and philosophical underpinning were at odds with many of the established ways of getting things done. At the outset of the programme, Warren ruffled feathers in particular at the World Health Organisation (WHO) by criticising the commendable but unobtainable goals for total primary health care for every human being (set out in a WHO declaration in 1978) and instead advocated a selective assault on those few diseases that caused the highest mortality among the world's poor.[50] In a similar fashion, he was also critical of the focus of the WHO's Tropical Diseases Research Programme (TDR), which he believed wrongly targeted diseases that did not cause the greatest suffering to the greatest number of people. Moreover, the GND sought to understand the mechanisms of disease by way of the use of molecular sciences, whereas the TDR's original mission was to use immunology to develop new tools and strategies to combat tropical diseases. Understandably then, there was some initial bureaucratic friction between the free enterprise ethos of the RF and the more politically sensitive WHO. However, resistance soon turned to (competitive) acceptance: Warren invested emotional capital each year by attending WHO meetings, and the GND and TDR programmes continued to run in parallel for a decade. Scott Halstead, Warren's colleague at the RF in the 1980s, concludes of their professional co-existence, "I think if you had gotten Ken in a reflective mood he would have said, 'No, TDR is a good thing.' After all, while the TDR diseases were fewer, they were many of the same ones that we were supporting."[51]

---

[47]Scott Halstead, personal communication.

[48]Sylvia Warren, personal communication.

[49]John Bruer, personal communication.

[50]Richard Peto, personal communication.

[51]Scott Halstead, personal communication.

There is little doubt that, building on the foundations laid by an earlier generation of scientists, the GND programme transformed parasitology from a lower technical endeavour to one that was at the forefront of the biotechnology revolution. And yet the GND was viewed by some as being peopled by "Johnny-come-latelies" with Warren evaluated alternatively as an "upstart" or a "new kid on the block."[52] These views may have evolved in response to the fact that the GND *was* indeed an exclusive club and was recognised as such by those both inside and outside its sphere of influence. Hans Wigzell was conscious of this situation and believed that it emanated from those who possibly felt threatened by microbiology and the new technologies that were being applied to the field. The rumblings from the establishment were subdued rather than overt, but they were unambiguously felt by Wigzell: "It was somehow that unless you had contracted malaria, or any other parasitic diseases yourself, or that you had been swinging in the jungle or been getting infected, you were not really a true person to be working in tropical diseases. I wouldn't call it vehement, but it was an *uppish* kind of treatment, with Ken treated like an underdog who was doing things that were 'not completely proper'."[53]

The disparaging view that Wigzell detected was not held by everyone. Bridget Ogilvie attended some of the GND meetings as an independent adjudicator and eschewed belligerence for a more balanced evaluation of Warren's contribution to neglected diseases: "I greatly admired and respected what Ken did—a lot of strengths in parasitology in the US now are because of Ken. But what I objected to with his GND was that everything that the Wellcome Trust or the MRC or anybody else funded, he took the credit for. He would give a group, who the Wellcome Trust was spending £1 million on, $50,000 or $100,000, and then take credit for everything that came out of it. I really objected to that. I thought it was beyond tolerance…."[54] This propensity to "big himself up" had been noted before. As a grant-maker, Warren was both entrepreneurial and enthusiastic. Kerr White, his Deputy Director at the RF, used to say that when a horse and rabbit stew was about to be made, Ken was there with his rabbit. But after the stew had been made, everyone believed that Ken had brought the horse.[55] Joe Cook had also encountered this exact phenomenon on several occasions; nonetheless, the sense of injustice was attenuated by the feeling that the investment had been shrewd of perception and profound in legacy: "Ken learned to use power very well, that was part of his genius, and when it came to funding schistosomiasis and the Molecular Parasitology Course at Woods Hole, I guess he probably did bring the rabbit and I brought the horse. But the course was very important for bringing people into parasitology research."[56] Even those who were outside the GND orbit were often

---

[52]Keith McAdam, personal communication.

[53]Hans Wigzell, personal communication.

[54]Dame Bridget Ogilvie, personal communication.

[55]John Bruer, personal communication.

[56]Joe Cook, personal communication.

quick to acknowledge the programme's strengths. In the 1970s, for instance, there were only two laboratories in the world working with cellular immunology on schistosomiasis: Ken Warren's in Cleveland and Dan Colley's in Nashville. Dan was not invited to be a part of the GND network and never attended any of their meetings, even though Ken Warren knew him well and had helped him at the beginning of his career. Inevitably Dan felt neglected and left out of the cama-raderie, spirit of optimism, and collective endeavour that defined the annual meetings. Nevertheless, he recognised the subtle link between the network's prodigious success and the human condition: "The reason people really liked the GND was the sense of *recognition*. Bringing scientists together and showing respect for what they do is important, because scientists don't often get that. That was probably the telling thing. Certainly, getting some money doesn't hurt, nor does meeting important people from other fields … but simply having a group to identify with is part of what I think it did."[57]

The GND programme forms an important chapter in the anthropology of tropical diseases. The interdisciplinary approach led to a great leap forward in under-standing pathogenesis and represented the first attempt to apply modern biomedical technology in the elucidation of the mechanisms of disease that were prevalent in developing countries. At the same time, it gave renewed vitality to parasitology and elevated the status of tropical medicine by developing new tools and methods for the control of what were the great neglected diseases.

As the architect of the GND network, Warren tried to pull off a difficult bal-ancing act: using modern, expensive molecular science developed in the West to bring a greater understanding of the diseases that were devastating the lives of the poorest people on the planet. This involved funding researchers at two of the world's leading centres of biomedical science, the University of Oxford and the Karolinska Institute, which inevitably led to accusations of elitism. Funds were paid directly to the respective institutions and then channeled to the specific groups. The first RF grant arrived in Sweden in September 1979, and the research unit consisted of two closely collaborating research teams within the Departments of Immunology at the University of Stockholm and the Karolinska Institute. The unit also worked in close association with the department of Medical Genetics (Uppsala University) and the Department of Infectious Diseases (Karolinska Institute). Certainly both Peter Perlmann and Hans Wigzell in Sweden were brilliant immunologists: Perlmann had particularly wide scientific interests, ranging from developmental biology to the importance of delineating the function of individual lymphocyte subsets and the co-operation of cells in understanding immunity. His recruitment into the GND marked a new, highly productive phase in his career in which he made contributions to the pathogenesis of cerebral malaria, whereas his department's training of a succession of doctoral students from malaria-endemic countries led him to become

---

[57]Dan Colley, personal communication.

a member of the Malaria Vaccine Steering Committee for many years.[58] GND
funding also transformed the fortunes and directions of the wider institutions, and
much of the seed-corn funding given by the RF continues to have a long-term
impact today. The creation of the Chair of Parasitology at the Karolinska Institute
was a direct consequence of Warren's programme: While looking at parasitic
research in his own country and across the other foundational units, Hans Wigzell
suggested that "seldom before has such relatively little money had such an impact
on the course of research in tropical medicine."[59] Meanwhile, in Oxford the RF's
funding came as a financial lifeline at a time when support for science in general,
and for work in the developing world in particular, had decreased in the UK. GND
support enabled Oxford medicine to develop enduring links with a number of
centres in the developing world: An encounter "over a good bottle of scotch" at the
inaugural GND meeting in New York between David Weatherall and the director of
the Wellcome Trust, Peter Williams, gave birth to a series of partnerships between
British universities and centres in the tropics.[60] This meeting led to the establishment of the Oxford–Wellcome Trust unit in Thailand in 1979 and began a programme that altered the concept of tropical medicine to medicine in the tropics.
This template was subsequently expanded to encompass partnerships in India,
Indonesia, Vietnam, Sri Lanka, Laos, and Jamaica. In addition to producing
international leaders in tropical medicine research, these connections led to
important developments in the management of common diseases such as malaria.
Weatherall's contribution to understanding the cause of thalassemia, and his life-
long contribution to the control of tropical diseases in poor countries, was recognised in 2010 when he was awarded the Lasker Prize.

Even those who criticised the GND's perceived elitism acknowledged that
Warren's selectivity was perhaps a necessary byproduct of the quest to attract the
best investigators and to supercharge the field. The immunologist Alan Sher spent
much of his scientific life at the NIH, and early in his training he was the beneficiary
of a Research Career Development Award in Geographic Medicine from the RF. At
the end of the 1980s, he perfectly captured the calibrated balance of forces and
interests that Warren recognised to be inherent but inescapable dichotomies of his
plans: "Although I have criticised the GND programme for its elitism in terms of
institutions and groups supported and neglect of talented investigators already in the
field of parasitology, its overall impact has been nothing short of outstanding. It has
helped to bring parasitology into the modern age, made it a fashionable subject for
the basic scientist, provided many investigators with a chance to enter the field and
helped launch their careers (e.g. myself)."[61] There is no doubt that Warren made the

---

[58]P. Perlmann in M. Coluzzi & D. Bradley, *Parasitologia. The Malaria Challenge after one hundred years of malariology*, Rome: Lombardo, 1999, p. 7.
[59]K. S. Warren & C. C. Jimenez (eds), *The Great Neglected Diseases of Mankind Biomedical Research Network: 1978–1988*. New York: The Rockefeller Foundation, 1988, p. 37.
[60]David Weatherall, personal communication.
[61]K. S. Warren & C. C. Jimenez (eds), *The Great Neglected Diseases of Mankind Biomedical Research Network: 1978–1988*. New York: The Rockefeller Foundation, 1988, p. 309.

careers of a generation of biomedical scientists in the US and across the world. John David, Hans Wigzell, Peter Perlmann, Michael Sela, James Kazura, Dick Guerrant, Adel Mahmoud, Gerald Keusch, Tony Cerami, Peter Hotez, Adolfo Martinez-Palomo, and many others were brought into the field of infectious diseases by the charm, vision, and sheer force of Warren's personality.

In 2014 an article in The Lancet, looking back at a century of the RF's existence, described the GND network as an example of its "excellent philanthropic work."[62] For a variety of reasons, Warren was a more influential figure than has generally been appreciated. His ideas were ahead of their time as he defined a new field of study and its lingua franca. Christopher Murray, now Director of the Health Institute for Health Metrics and Evaluation in Seattle, met Warren in the mid-1980s and recognises that his concepts still have a resonance today: "I think the GND programme had a great effect. He coined the term and it has stuck, and now people compete to call their disease 'neglected.' There is [now] a bit of a war about what the borders are, what is in and what is not. Is leprosy neglected? Is rabies? There are a lot of different definitions of what is neglected, and I think that the concept can reasonably be traced back to Ken."[63]

As well as taking the field in a new direction, Ken Warren's aim was for the GND to make a major impact on reducing the burden of disease while at the same time infusing young scientists with the immense importance, fascination, and potential of tropical disease research. For many investigators, meeting Ken Warren was a turning point in their lives that took them in new, previously unimagined destinations. One such scientist was Gerald "Jerry" Keusch, a former Director of the Fogarty International Centre for Global Health at the NIH and a world-renowned researcher in tropical diseases. After securing a grant for a decade from the GND, he then followed it up with a further 10-year grant from the RF, which was used to establish a partnership with the Christian Medical College in Vellore, India, which itself became a leading infectious-disease center. Jerry recognised that Warren had great skill at creating programmes and mobilizing money but also that he was greatly admired by the cadre of young scientists who had been so carefully selected. Warren created an environment where highly competitive research scientists in the real world could lower the antenna and interact in a collective way: "At the annual meetings, everybody participated, and you wanted to present your best work. There was a true sense of collaboration. I have not seen that in any other group that I've been part of. I think that most of us who were there would say that that period of time was probably the best in our scientific career. Ken's legacy is the network itself. We metastasised and spawned a new revolution in tropical diseases; it goes from the very molecular, upstream, down to the delivery of health care and health

[62]L. C. Chen, "China Medical Board: a century of Rockefeller health philanthropy," *The Lancet*, 384: 717–719, 2014.

[63]Christopher Murray, personal communication.

care systems. That has really come out of the drive that Ken imparted to it. It is quite remarkable."[64]

In addition to the benefits envisaged and hoped for, the GND had many unforeseen positive influences. In Oxford, for instance, the GND legacy helped to influence research in tropical medicine to the more general benefit of the subject: attracting excellent young clinicians into the field, both from the UK and from the developing world, stimulating undergraduates to spend elective periods in the Third World, and leading to the establishment of an undergraduate teaching programme in tropical medicine. It also had a major influence on the format of the Oxford Textbook of Medicine, which, probably more than any other standard medical textbook, deals with problems in the developing world.

The GND was not the sole focus of Warren's activities at the RF. In 1977, when he was appointed Director of Health Sciences, he was responsible for distributing $100 million over a decade in three major areas: In addition to biomedical research by way of the GND, he also was responsible for the development of the International Clinical Epidemiological Network (INCLEN) and the creation of efficient, low-cost medical- and health-information systems. These new challenges would require all of Warren's drive, ingenuity, salesmanship, and passion to make them succeed. One momentous undertaking that had been incubating for many years came to the fore in the early 1980s: the campaign to immunise the world's poorest children against killer diseases. Warren knew the field well, having helped to establish the WHO's Programme for Vaccine Development and their Scientific Advisory Group of Experts (SAGE). In the words of his colleague, Scott Halstead, "'vaccines' was every other word that came out of Ken's mouth."[65] Overlapping with, and leading on from, the GND era, vaccines were to be Warren's next great project.

---

[64]Gerald Keusch, personal communication.

[65]Scott Halstead, personal communication.

Chapter 3
Selective Primary Healthcare

The ideological differences concerning the most effective way to prevent and treat tropical diseases originate from two of the Victorian founding fathers of the specialty, Sir Patrick Manson and Sir Donald Ross. The dynamics of the personal relationship that existed between these highly influential nineteenth century physicians was at times neuralgic.[1] The experiences of these two pioneering investigators with the microscope—still an essential instrument for investigators in the tropics today—and with providing medical care in the tropics divided the field into two opposing camps. For Manson, who discovered the mosquito transmission of filariasis—the cause of elephantiasis—in Amoy, China, in the 1870s, salvation for European colonisers of the tropics lay in the hard science of the laboratory. In the 1898 preface to his book, *Tropical Diseases*: *A Manual of the Diseases of Warm Climates*, he outlined the imperial way forward: "I now firmly believe in the possibility of tropical colonisation by the white races. Heat and moisture are not in themselves the direct causes of any important tropical disease. The direct causes of 99% of these diseases are germs. To kill them is simply a matter of knowledge." Conversely, for Ross, Britain's first Nobel laureate for discovering that the mosquito was the vector for malaria, it was a more holistic approach that would help to bring the ambrosia of well-being, the vital elements of which were "general living conditions, diet, and sanitation as the main determinants of health." This marked the beginning of a polarisation of approaches to health in the less developed world that still persisted when Warren began his career in international medicine: Could, and should, disease be alleviated simply through the application of science and medicine, or was a more effective route found in improving wider social conditions?

By the early part of the twentieth century, the Manson and Ross methodologies had been distilled into the so-called "vertical" approaches—direct, targeted pro-

---

[1]M. Worboys, "The emergence of tropical medicine: a study in the establishment of a scientific speciality", in G. Lemaine (ed.), *Perspectives on the emergence of scientific disciplines*, The Hague: Mouton, 1976.

© Springer International Publishing AG 2017
C. Keating, *Kenneth Warren and the Great Neglected Diseases*
of Mankind Programme, Springer Biographies,
DOI 10.1007/978-3-319-50147-5_3

grammes using specific technologies such as drugs, vaccines, and insecticides—and "horizontal" approaches, which simultaneously used all means—medical, ecological, sociological, and political—to improve health; the former strategy gained ascendancy.

One of the first such large-scale vertical attempts to deal with rampant ill health in tropical regions was the RF's campaign of 1913 to eradicate hookworms, which debilitate hundreds of millions of people across the globe. Practically all parasitic illnesses are diseases of poverty, and the long-term answer to their control is to eliminate poverty rather than develop biomedical tools or intervention policies. However, tools such as drugs and vaccines can complement efforts to reduce poverty or can at least alleviate some suffering in the absence of poverty reduction.[2] The Rockefeller campaign began in the southern United States and was then continued in 6 continents, 52 countries, and 29 islands. Ultimately the campaign failed because of the enormous reproductive potential of the worms, each capable of producing 20,000 eggs per day, coupled with the lack of highly effective nontoxic drugs and the inadequacy of sanitary facilities.[3]

Although "vertical" approaches to the treatment of tropical diseases remained popular, they had similar problems to the hookworm campaign. The WHO's initial eradication programmes in the 1950s onward were dominated by mass campaigns against tuberculosis, yaws, and malaria aided by the therapeutic invention of penicillin, streptomycin, and other pharmaceutical advances. Yaws, a crippling, disfiguring disease primarily affecting the skin and bones, is caused by *Treponema pallidum* subspecies *pertenue*. Using injections of penicillin to treat the diseases, the yaws-control programme typified the vertical approach that Manson outlined half a century previously, and its initial success made it an outlier for a more ambitious undertaking as the WHO moved on to tackle the eradication of malaria.[4] This process of accelerating the application of biomedical science to Third World problems began to lose momentum, however, when the massive global malaria eradication effort, begun in 1955, collapsed in dystopian disarray in the 1970s. It would have been hard to predict that the efforts of the newly created WHO Expert Committee on Malaria, which acted as the intellectual powerhouse for the attempt at eradicating the disease, would end in the chaos of the 1980s when research work

---

[2]M. Tanner & D. Evans, "Vaccines or Drugs: Complementarity is Crucial." *Parasitology Today*, vol. 10, no. 10, p. 406, 1994.

[3]This said, the campaign was more effective in the southeastern US during the 1920s because the prevalence of hookworm decreased markedly. This may have been due to the vigorous education programme that accompanied the treatment or a general upswing in the area's economy. See G. W. Esch, *Parasites and Infectious Disease Discovery by Serendipity, and Otherwise*. CUP, 2007, p. 228.

[4]Chris Murray, personal communication. By the end of 1964, the prevalence of yaws had reduced from 50 million to 2.5 million cases—see G. M. Antal & G. Causse, "The control of endemic treponematoses." *Rev Infect Dis*; 7 Suppl. 2: S220-6, 1985.

on malaria was avoided.[5] Nearly $4 billion had been spent on malaria eradication, but environmental changes and interventions had led the malaria parasite and its vector to develop resistance to drugs and insecticides. The disease had evolved and thus was not the static entity of the past. The failure to fulfill the promise to eradicate malaria led to a wholesale revolt—not from the poor, who were increasingly subject to the ravages of the disease, but from the scientific community and the WHO in particular—against the strategy of disease eradication and the vertical approach in general. Disenchantment was so great that even the total and unprecedented success of the smallpox-eradication programme, which was achieved in 1979, had virtually no effect in rehabilitating the centrality of science to health amelioration.

Unsurprisingly, with so many diseases being manifestations of poverty, horizontal approaches became more prominent as the backlash developed. In the period from 1965 to the early 1980s, many within the institutions of world health saw socio-economic development as an answer to the entire developing world's diseases. The change in emphasis corresponded to the reconfiguration of agencies that were the custodians of the world's most vulnerable populations. With some 3 billion people in those countries having infectious diseases, it was imperative to reduce the sequence of exposure, disability, and death. The abandonment of the disease-targeted, vertical approach led to a preoccupation with primary health care, which was defined "in its original and narrowest sense (as) frontline or first-contact care, where people meet health workers."[6]

The doctrine of comprehensive primary health care was nurtured by the evangelical Halfdan T. Mahler, who was appointed the director general of WHO in May 1973. Mahler, a Dane, came from a missionary background, an antecedent that permeated his thinking. The son of a Baptist minister, he believed that health for all was a fundamental human right. In addition, like Warren, he was charismatic and persuasive. Unlike his colleague, however, Mahler strongly favoured the increasingly fashionable "horizontal" approach to disease control. His, and by extension the WHO's attitude toward immunisation, was in part due to the failure of the malaria programmes but also due to a profound shift in philosophy. Mahler had trained in public health and specialised in tuberculosis and had then worked on mass campaigns in South America and India that he had come to dislike. Under Mahler's leadership, the WHO experienced a metamorphosis, a philosophical redirection away from curative toward preventive care.[7] For Mahler, the most productive way forward was to jettison the white heat of medical technology being promoted by top physicians and bureaucrats and embrace the ideal of primary

---

[5]M. Coluzzi & D. Bradley, *Parasitologia. The Malaria Challenge after one hundred years of malariology*, Rome: Lombardo, 1999, p. 16.

[6]G. Walt & P. Vaughan, An introduction to primary health care approach in developing countries: a review with selected annotated references. London: Ross Institute of Tropical Hygiene publ. no. 13, 1981.

[7]J. Goodfield, *A Chance to Live*: *The heroic story of the global campaign to immunise the world's children*, Macmillan, New York, 1990, p. 3.

health workers based on the celebrated barefoot doctors of 1920s China. His analysis was heartfelt, and at the 1976 World Health Assembly, Mahler proposed the goal of "Health for All by the Year 2000." To achieve such a noble objective would take unwavering persistence, but for Mahler the status quo was untenable: "Many social evolutions and revolutions have taken place because the social structures were crumbling. There are signs that the scientific and technical structures of public health are also crumbling."[8]

The deeply held religious beliefs that informed Mahler's thinking led him to seek an Edenic solution to the diseases that disproportionately affected the world's poor. Just such an opportunity to realise his vision occurred in September 1978, when an International Conference on Primary Health Care was held at Alma-Ata, then the capital of the Soviet Republic of Kazakhstan located in the foothills of the Trans-Ili Alatau Mountains. The 6-day meeting was jointly sponsored by the WHO and UNICEF and was attended by 3000 delegates from 134 governments across the world. The culmination of the ambitious conference was marked by the production of the Declaration of Alma-Ata, which enshrined health as "a fundamental human right." The means of achieving this commendable aim was through comprehensive primary health care, which was defined as being "the attainment by all peoples of the world by the year 2000 of a level of health that will permit them to lead a socially and economically productive life. Primary health care is the key to attaining this target... [and] includes at least: education concerning prevailing health problems and the methods of preventing and controlling them; promotion of food supply and proper nutrition, an adequate supply of safe water and basic sanitation; maternal and child health care, including family planning; immunisation against the major infectious diseases; prevention and control of locally endemic diseases; appropriate treatment of common diseases and injuries; the provision of essential drugs."[9]

From the outset, the Declaration of Alma-Ata was seen as controversial, particularly in its utopian definition of health—taken from the WHO constitution of 1948, i.e., "a state of complete physical, mental, and social well-being and not merely the absence of disease or infirmity"—and its strategy and timetable under which such conditions would come about. Mahler's altruism expressed itself in the need to help the forward march of human beings both economically and socially. Idealism is almost always a good thing; it can bring clarity, define goals, and power dreams; yet there is an obligation to harness its emancipative forces to political realities if it is not to become a hindrance. For Warren, Mahler's Alma-Ata epistle, while noble and portentous, was also a utopian chimera, a distraction from finding the most efficient way of improving the life expectancy and reducing the suffering of the world's poorest people. Instead, Warren advocated against the popular grain, and continued to ascribe to the Harvard microbiologist Geoffrey Edsall's classical

---

[8]M. Cueto, "The Origins of Primary Health Care and Selective Primary Health Care." American Journal of Public Health. Vol. 44. No 11, p. 3, 2004.

[9]*Primary Health Care*. A Joint Report by the Director-General of the World Health Organisation and the Executive Director of the United Nations Children's Fund. WHO: New York, 1978.

statement, made in 1963, that "never in the history of human progress has a better and cheaper method of preventing illness been developed than immunisation at its best."[10] Starting first at Case Western, and then as Director of Health Sciences at the Rockefeller Foundation, Warren had set himself the task of designing a strategy to reduce the burden of ill health that disproportionately affected children; living in the temperate regions between the Tropics of Capricorn and Cancer. Warren was not naïve and recognised that many of the problems underlying the prevalence of tropical diseases were primarily social, economic, and geopolitical in nature. Nevertheless, in his mind, "vertical" approaches that targeted specific killer diseases, very often by way of vaccination programmes, would prove to be the best short-term method of eradicating tropical diseases, even if the longer-term panacea remained the wider alleviation of social poverty.

Warren was not alone in this thinking. Tore Godal, the Norwegian immunologist and champion of international health initiates, also viewed the policy of comprehensive primary health care as unrealistically paradisiacal. Godal's own career was guided not by a sense of idealism, but more by a combination of curiosity and adventure, which was inspired in him as a child by his mother's ethereal fairy tales of audacity and daring. As a young researcher in the 1970s, Godal worked on leprosy in Ethiopia and is a reliable interpreter of the Alma-Ata era in global health: "It was a kind of romantic ideal based on the barefoot doctors, [whereby] a primary health care worker would have a month of training but then when you saw the list of what the person was to undertake, it was something like 30 different courses, so it was totally unrealistic. It was ideological, idealistic [in the] context that it would never work in terms of making it successful."[11]

Sceptics, such as Godal, were far keener on the idea for *selective* primary health care devised by Ken Warren, a strategy that emerged from a Bellagio conference on "Health, population and development" in April 1979. Warren organised the meeting, and his boss at the RF, John Knowles, gave the keynote address in which he emphasised the central totemic principle that applied to policy options within the health sector, namely, "those that will succeed."[12] At the meeting, Warren—in collaboration with Julia Walsh, who was then a visiting research fellow at the RF—presented a ground-breaking paper, which in its evidence-based approach and advocacy of low-cost, high-impact medical technologies challenged the philosophy that underpinned Alma-Ata. In 1979, Walsh and Warren's paper "Selective primary health care: an interim strategy for disease control in developing countries" was published in the *New England Journal of Medicine*. The article marked a departure from the traditional indicators, such as life expectancy at birth and infant mortality, to look at specific causes of death. In the paper, the major infectious diseases of the

---

[10]J. H. L. Playfair, in I. M. Roitt (ed.), *Immune Intervention: New Trends in Vaccines*, vol 1., Academic Press, 1984, p. 1.

[11]Tore Godal, personal communication.

[12]J. H. Knowles, "Health, population and development." *Soc. Sci. Med.* 14C, 67, 1980.

less developed world were placed in the order of their importance based on the number of deaths produced, and the disabilities caused, ranging from weakness and inability to work and learn to crippling and disfigurement.[13] This exercise had never been performed before, and it showed that the two most devastating health problems in the developing world were diarrheal diseases and respiratory infections of infants and young children, each of which was responsible for 5 to 10 million deaths per year. Other major diseases cited were malaria, measles, schistosomiasis, whooping cough, tuberculosis, tetanus, and diphtheria. The authors advocated "instituting selective primary health care directed at preventing or treating those few diseases responsible for the greatest mortality in less developed areas and for which interventions of proven high efficacy exist."[14] The aberrant article outlined a cost-effective and workable strategy for the control of "killer" diseases that would save the lives of millions of children each year. These recommended *vertical* measures were immunisation against tuberculosis, polio, measles, diphtheria, whooping cough, and tetanus; the use in patients with diarrhoea of oral rehydration therapy; the treatment of life-threatening malaria; and the breast-feeding of infants, which provides the child with protective antibodies present in a mother's milk. This phased approach to the introduction of primary health care was an unconcealed acknowledgement that the WHO's objective "Health for All by 2000" was unattainable, a belief that Warren and Walsh bolstered by quoting on the opening page of their article the president of the World Bank, Robert S. McNamara, who in his 1978 annual report had drawn attention to financial realities that made the WHO's wholly admirable strategy untenable: "Even if the projected—and optimistic—growth rates in the developing world are achieved, some 600 million individuals at the end of the century will remain trapped in absolute poverty. Absolute poverty is a condition of life so characterised by malnutrition, illiteracy, disease, high infant mortality, and low life expectancy as to be beneath any reasonable definition of human decency (Fig. 3.1)."[15]

Perhaps unsurprisingly, the paper provoked widespread criticism and led Warren to later reflect that "in retrospect, Walsh and I realised that we had unwittingly entered directly into the great debate on vertical versus horizontal health interventions."[16] A great debate took place within the *New England Journal of Medicine*, with some of the disapproval at Walsh and Warren's targeted programme being more a question of emphasis than outright indignation. Some disagreed with "the priority ranking according to a number of disease-control activities," whereas

---

[13]K. S. Warren, 'The Alma-Ata Declaration: *Health for All by the Year 2000? Britannica Book of the Year*, Encyclopedia Britannica, Inc. (Chicago, 1990), p. 7.

[14]J. A. Walsh & K. S. Warren, "Selective primary health care: an interim strategy for disease control in developing countries." New Engl J Med; 301, p. 967, 1979.

[15]J. A. Walsh & K. S. Warren, "Selective primary health care: an interim strategy for disease control in developing countries." New Engl J Med; 301, p. 967, 1979.

[16]K. S. Warren, 'The Alma-Ata Declaration: *Health for All by the Year 2000? Britannica Book of the Year*, Encyclopedia Britannica, Inc. (Chicago, 1990), p. 7.

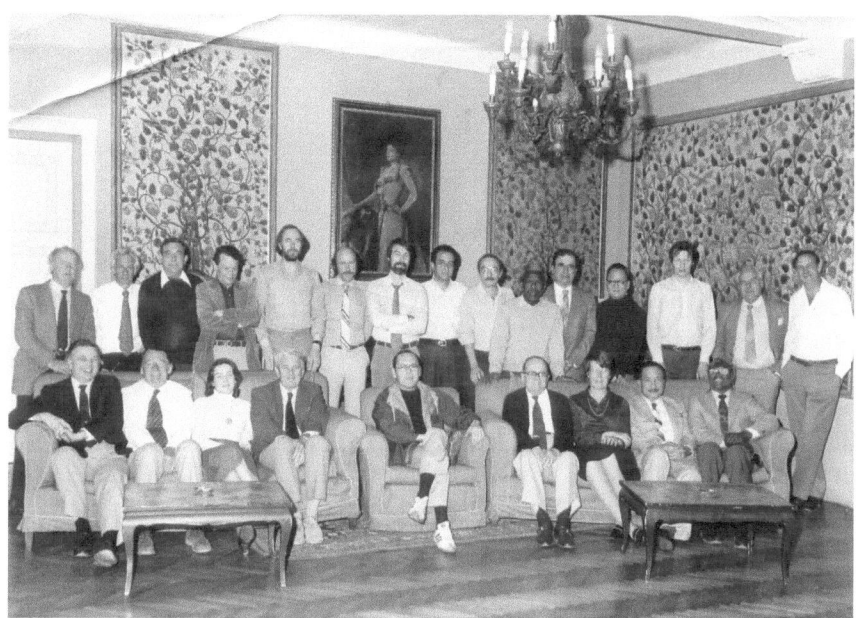

Fig. 3.1 Bellagio conference on Health and Population in Development, April, 1979. The theme of the conference was helminths, with a particular emphasis on schistosomiasis. The scientific meeting had an emphasis on funding, reflected in the presence of representatives from the RF, WHO and Wellcome Trust. Standing. *Left* to *right*, George Nelson, John David, Andre Capron (Pasteur Institute, Lille), Peter Perlmann (Karolinska Institute), Graham Mitchell (6th) (WEHI), Adolfo Martinez-Palomo (8th) (National Polytechnic Institute, Mexico) Peter Williams (15th) (Wellcome Trust Director). Sitting. *Left* to *right*, Ruth Arnon (3rd) (Weizmann Institute of Science), *centre* a regal looking Ken Warren, Bridget Ogilvie (7th) (Wellcome Trust), and Adetokunbo Lucas (9th) (WHO-TDR). Courtesy of Christopher Warren

others believed that "any attempt at improving health in the developing world must address the social and economic conditions that lead to poor health.[17] In reply, Walsh and Warren took a conciliatory, realistic, and actuarial stance: "Selective primary health care must be as simple as possible while being flexible and sensitive to the needs of the people, but the bottom line is a significant reduction in morbidity and mortality at an affordable cost; the alternatives in many areas of the world are either thinly spread, ineffective programmes or nothing."[18] This did not prevent the concept of *selective* primary health care becoming anathema to a broad group of primary health care protagonists.[19] Chris Murray summed up the seemingly

---

[17]R. H. Henderson & J. Keja, "Letter to the Editor", N Engl J Med; 302: 757–759, 27 March 1980; D. Campos-Outcalt, "Letter to the Editor", N Engl J Med; 302: 757–759, 27 March 1980.

[18]J. A. Walsh & K. S. Warren, "Letter to the Editor", N Engl J Med; 302: 757–759, 27 March 1980.

[19]David Bradley, personal communication.

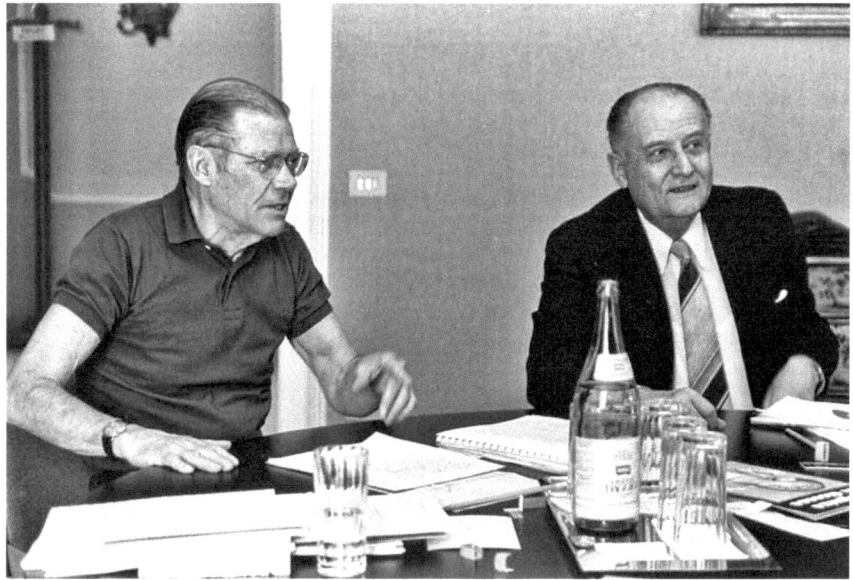

Fig. 3.2 On the *left*, Robert McNamara, at the time, President of the World Bank. Courtesy of Christopher Warren

intractable positions succinctly: "Selective health care was a very controversial paper; there was the WHO view and the Walsh and Warren view, and it was where two worlds collided (Fig. 3.2)."[20]

David Bradley, one of the world's leading communicable disease epidemiologists and for 30 years the Professor of Tropical Hygiene at the LSHTM, also took issue with some aspects of Walsh and Warren's work. Because of their shared interest in helminthology, Bradley had on the one hand great admiration for Warren's campaigning ability to elevate parasitology within the iconography of international health and to mobilise funds. He recognised that although "Ken did a good job," this did not prevent him from observing that, "he also had an astounding ego—and I would step on it occasionally."[21] However, he was also uncomfortable with the self-promotional side of American science, which, to him, Warren typified. Bradley preferred the more understated classical British approach as long as it didn't transmogrify into an inverted form of snobbery. Moreover, Bradley suspected that Warren had mistakenly inflated the harm caused by schistosomiasis in the 1979 paper and elsewhere.[22] Warren had spent much of his scientific life—at the NIH and CWRU—investigating schistosomiasis, seeing it as a disease that was

---

[20]Chris Murray, personal communication.

[21]David Bradley, personal communication.

[22]David Bradley, personal communication.

both neglected and its burden misjudged. From David Bradley's perspective, the mathematical underpinning of the 1979 NEJM paper was questionable, and he believed that Julia Walsh, who had studied at the LSHTM, should have "learned what we taught her." Indeed, although it is true that most infectious disease epidemiologists now accept that Warren overstated the mortality of the disease, he may well have underestimated the long-term morbidity levels resulting from schistosomiasis.[23]

Although Warren and Walsh were co-authors of the paper, the relationship between the two could more accurately be described as mentor and protégé. Yet when it came to the allocation of blame for undermining the Alma-Ata declaration, the liability was shared equally. Julia Walsh believed that "the WHO hated Ken," while she herself remembers being reproached by Bradley (Walsh had recently gained her MSc in tropical public health at the LSHTM), who said, "What did we teach you? Did we teach you Alma-Ata so that you could write an article like this?" In Walsh's own words, the paper was "enormously controversial."[24]

What wasn't tendentious about the Walsh and Warren analysis was the logic of their numerical approach, which foreshadowed the *World Development Report: Investing in Health*, which was funded by the World Bank, published in 1993.[25] With a team led by Dean Jamison and containing, among others, Christopher Murray and Richard Feachem, this iconic report used the "disability-adjusted life year" to measure the burden of disease. This enabled the authors to give a cost–benefit analysis without putting a dehumanising cash-value on a human life. As the 1993 report stated on its opening page, "In addition to premature mortality, a substantial portion of the burden of disease consists of disability, ranging from polio-related paralysis to blindness to suffering brought about by severe psychosis. To measure the burden of disease, this Report uses the disability-adjusted life year (DALY), a measure that combines healthy life years lost because of premature mortality with those lost as a result of disability."[26] In doing so, mortality and morbidity were combined in a single common metric in an attempt to quantify the two components in much the same way as Walsh and Warren had performed. Julia Walsh has no doubt that "unquestionably, Selective Primary Health Care was a precursor to the use of DALYs in the 1993 World Bank Report. On many different

---

[23]Dan Colley, personal communication.

[24]Julia Walsh, personal communication.

[25]Another highly influential precursor of the DALYs was a paper by P. Smith, K. P. Nimo et al. as the "Ghana Health Assessment Project Team" in Int. J. Epidemiology 10: 73–80, 1981, for developing-country use. This group introduced the concept of "amount of health life lost", combining measures of the effects of a disease, in terms of life lost both from mortality (expected years of life remaining had the disease not occurred) and from morbidity (severity and duration of disability). What was particularly distinctive according to Peter Smith, "was the group's attempt to assign specific weights to different kinds of disability." DALYs are calculated by combining the years of life lost (YLL) from premature mortality with the years of life lived with disability (YLD), weighted according to severity grading. Thus DALY = YLL + YLD.

[26]World Development Report 1993: Investing in Health, OUP, 1993, p. 1.

occasions during the preparation, Dean Jamison, Chris Murray, and other authors referred to the paper as the first time someone had tried to quantify mortality and morbidity from many causes to understand their relative importance. Because of the paper, the authors understood the power of quantifying the cause of death and disability."[27] It was now going to be possible to evaluate the cost of such diverse health components as an air ambulance or an educational campaign highlighting the public health dangers of drinking dirty water. For some within the highest echelons of the great international agencies, the World Bank report finally managed to make selective primary health care respectable.[28]

From personal experience, Warren knew only too well that health priorities in the developing world, and in the developed world for that matter, were simply not set in any systematic manner. As a consequence, a litany of notorious aberrations occurred across the globe including the South Asian nation that declared leprosy and tuberculosis as its two major health priorities while its children were dying due to diarrheal and respiratory infections and the West African country whose main concern was whether to do coronary bypass operations in the capital city or send patients abroad rather than tackling intractable problems of nutrition and starvation. For Warren, allowing politicians and bureaucrats to set health objectives was equally reckless as they would be subservient to the sectional interests of family, party, or community. Nor did he expect salvation to come from his own profession because "most physicians lack the knowledge of epidemiology, statistics, and economics required for priority setting, having been trained largely in the tertiary health care facilities with a primary focus on rare, advanced, and fatal diseases."[29] Warren's most vehement criticism, however, was directed at the WHO for what he believed was an abrogation of their responsibilities by setting "horizontal" priorities at Alma-Ata and their advocacy of an amorphous manifesto for health that failed to target the most important killer diseases in a rational fashion. Instead, Walsh and Warren showed how to decipher the components of the morbidity and mortality rates in the developing world, and to determine priorities based on prevalence of disease, morbidity, and mortality. The bottom line was sacrosanct: Based on these criteria, a cost-effective means of preventing and controlling the selected diseases would be found.

This represented an experimental advance in efforts to systematise the establishment of priorities for the control of the major diseases in the developing world. Warren took a numerical view of world health, believing that arithmetic and the application of statistical methods were the best philosophy for setting health priorities, thus adhering to Major Greenwood's aphorism of a generation before, i.e., "medicine with the tears wiped off." Warren's case, made in his trademark flamboyant and unsubtle fashion, had a polarising effect at the WHO. This was at a time

---

[27]Julia Walsh, personal communication.

[28]David Bradley, personal communication.

[29]K. S. Warren, "The difficult art, science and politics of setting health priorities." *The Lancet*, 27 August 1988, pp. 498–499.

when the WHO was much more central in international health than it is today, and Warren proved to be an irritant, a pebble in the shoe of health politics, by asking awkward, uncomfortable questions: What are the priorities? What really matters? Where should resources go? The British epidemiologist Richard Peto, a renowned advocate of big numbers, worked with and was influenced by Warren and saw at first-hand the value of Warren's actions: "A lot of people were absolutely outraged that he should question the value of their programmes as to whether some other things should take precedent. He was saying 'well, what is the evidence on numbers? How many deaths are from this, and what can you do with the interventions that you're trying out?' He ruffled a lot of feathers at WHO, very definitely, but they needed to be."[30]

Warren had a good deal of immunity to the outrage that was directed against him. As seen with the GND programme, there was a single-mindedness about him that sometimes blinded him to the sensibilities of others, and that could create enmities both within the RF and the world outside. Although many would testify that Warren didn't mind causing turbulence, they might also feel that he didn't deliberately set out to do so or perhaps that he just didn't notice. It was merely a function of his enthusiasm and drive. The American epidemiologist, William "Bill" Foege, worked closely with Warren for many years witnessing his many heartfelt enthusiasms: "Ken was like a manic depressive, who was never depressive, he was just always manic and excited about everything. You know, Ken reminded me of a little boy in many ways, his enthusiasm was part of that—it was hard to get him down. The bigger the challenge, the more ideas he had on what could be performed to solve the problem. So, he's the type of person you like to see in global health that doesn't get beaten down, but just turns up every morning with new optimism."[31]

Now seen as a more influential figure than has generally been appreciated, Warren's dedication to large-scale implementation and his questioning of established theories caused huge interest as well indignation, and the 1979 paper proved to have a "massive impact" on subsequent global health policy.[32] As discussed previously, Warren and Walsh's advocacy of targeted assaults on specific diseases, and of a metric that could be used by donors, governments, and bilateral agencies for measuring impact, led directly to Dean Jamison's 1993 *World Development Report*. For Jamison, the affinity with Warren was based on a shared psychology: He believed they saw the world in similar ways. He was hugely persuaded by Warren's "vertical" interventions concentrating on diseases that could be addressed by technology. The World Bank report of 1993 is rightly celebrated as a major contribution to finding the most cost-effective form of medical intervention to help reduce the sequence of exposure, disability, and death in the developing world. After the report had been written, Jamison was invited to a meeting with his new boss, Michael Bruno. At the meeting, Bruno told his colleague, "You went into this

[30]Sir Richard Peto, personal communication.
[31]William Foege, personal communication.
[32]Julia Walsh, personal communication.

report pretty well knowing what your conclusions were going to be, I bet. I don't want to know what those conclusions were. I want to know what conclusion you came to that *wasn't* on that list." Jamison's answer was immediate: "Scientific advance rather than economic advance, and that [the] huge changes to human health over the century were a product of … technological change."[33] The recognition that the most important element driving improvements in health was scientific research was a vindication of Warren's beliefs, and so the decade-long controversy that had pursued Selective Primary Health Care like a recalcitrant meme ended with the widespread acceptance of its methodology.

The influence of Warren's belief in providing a solid financial basis for health research and development thus continues today and, according to his former collaborator, Julia Walsh, has "saved millions of children's lives."[34] Similar linkages and influences can be seen in Christopher Murray's *Global Burden of Disease* initiative.[35] While he was a young student (Doctor of Philiosphy) at Oxford, Murray had read Warren's *Good Health at Low Cost*, a publication that made many similar suggestions for the methodology of disease intervention as had the 1979 paper.[36] He remembers that "I needed some money to carry out my own study of comparing countries with the same level of health spending and had either good or bad levels of health provision. I wanted to do a good-health-care-at-low-cost study a bit more rigorously. So I wrote to Ken he said 'yes' and the Rockefeller paid for my DPhil fieldwork. So I picked pairs of countries that seemed to have similar levels of health spending and had either good or bad health at that level of spending, but were geographically similar in size or other aspects. I looked at three pairs of countries and spent three months in each country. I didn't come up with any great answers, but I got very interested in TB. Good health at low cost is the basis of what we do."[37] Thus, a distinct line of historical continuity is discernible between Warren and Murray, with the latter now in the vanguard of the movement dedicated to reducing long-term infant mortality and the global burden of disease.

---

[33]Dean Jamison, personal communication.

[34]Julia Walsh, personal communication.

[35]The first Global Burden of Disease study was published in 2010 and is recognised as the most authoritative work on the causes of ill health. One hundred eight countries are included in the Global Burden of Disease study, and the work takes in data from 1990 up to 2013.

[36]S. B. Halstead, J. A. Walsh & K. S. Warren (eds), *Good Health at Low Cost: Proceedings of a Conference at the Bellagio Conference Centre, Italy. 29 April – 3 May 1985*. New York: Rockefeller Foundation, 1985. The publication followed a meeting at Bellagio organised by Warren to bring together demographers, economists, and epidemiologists to examine why it was that some countries provided better health care than others while having similar levels of health expenditure. The study undermined the widely held belief that economic growth was a prerequisite for health improvement by making people aware that three of the poorest areas in the world— China, Sri Lanka, and India's Kerala State—had life expectancies of 65 years. It also underscored the benefits of expanding the application of existing knowledge and technologies in the Third World.

[37]Christopher Murray, personal communication.

During this period, two other connected issues continued to cause tension between Warren and the international health establishment. First, he was seen by some alternately as a representative of neo-liberalism and the private enterprise sector of health, a "new kid on the block, an upstart," and too unorthodox in his thinking.[38] Second, in 1975 the WHO had already established its Tropical Diseases Research Programme (TDR) with the following statement: "The recent enormous extension of knowledge in the biomedical sciences has as yet hardly begun to be applied to the problems of tropical diseases where methods of control and treatment have scarcely changed in the past 30 years."[39] With Warren launching the GND just 2 years later, one would have imagined that he was a wholehearted supporter of the TDR, but the reality was far from it. The programme involved five parasitic diseases—malaria, trypanosomiasis, leishmaniasis, schistosomiasis, and filariasis— and one bacterial disease, leprosy. However, rather like his later criticisms of the Alma-Ata Declaration, Warren was critical of the fact that the TDR's disease selection did not include diarrhea or pneumonia or even neonatal deaths.[40] Instead, Warren wanted the things that affected very large numbers of people to be taken appropriately seriously. The Thai biochemist, Yongyuth Yuthavong, was one of the GND's foundation heads, and today he is the Deputy Prime Minister of Thailand. In the 1970s, he worked on the basic aspect and biochemistry of malaria, and in addition to receiving grants from Warren, also had support from the TDR. He gives this nuanced insight into the feeling of disgruntlement: "I was amused and disturbed that Ken was so antagonistic to the TDR; he could be unkind to people and organisations. He was not convinced that WHO could do very much in achieving science. He [saw it] as being too much involved in global politics, so that real science had been neglected."[41] This observation was a distillation of the very profound differences between the WHO and Warren about the value and role of basic and western science in the developing world.

Following the outcry over the 1979 paper, Warren was more determined than ever to use his catalytic power to elevate children's wellbeing to the top of the international health agenda. This resolution was strengthened by the unfolding failure of the WHO's Expanded Programme of Immunisation (EPI), which had been launched in 1974. This was a targeted "vertical" initiative established the year after Mahler had become the WHO's director general. The immunisation programme, which included six infant vaccinations against diphtheria, pertussis, tetanus, poliomyelitis, measles, and tuberculosis, got off to a slow start with only 5% of children in the developing world being immunised by the end of the rollout

---

[38]Keith McAdam, personal communication.

[39]World Health Organisation. Tropical diseases today – the challenge and the opportunity. Geneva: World Health Organisation, 1975.

[40]Tore Godal was the Director of TDR from 1986 to 1998, and one of the reasons for the selection of leprosy may have been because he acted as a consultant to Howard Goodman, the first Director of TDR, 1973–74. From there he was chosen to be the head of a 3-year pilot project on leprosy in Ethiopia.

[41]Yongyuth Yuthavong, personal communication.

year.[42] The obstacles were more subtle and intractable than those of technology or money; they reflected (1) insufficient political will; (2) lack of both trained people and effective delivery systems for an immunisation protocol that required mothers and children to pay three visits to the health centres; (3) the problems of side effects of some vaccines; and (4) the fact that in developing countries, as in developed ones, curing diseases still took priority over preventing them.

Warren continued to be concerned about the number of these children that died or were crippled, blinded, or disabled from diseases that were preventable through immunisation. Averting their avoidable suffering and death became his *raison d'etre*. The opportunity to take further action arose on the morning of May 22 1983 when Jonas Salk walked into Warren's office at the RF's headquarters on the Avenue of the Americas. Salk had developed the first safe and effective vaccine for polio.[43] Moreover, he shared Warren's misgivings about the WHO's EPI, which by this time had been underway for almost a decade. Although the programme was high in quality, it was low in coverage, having immunised only approximately 10–15% of susceptible infants in the developing world. Salk wanted Warren's support in his campaign to get the inactivated polio vaccine (IPV) used in a global programme and believed that a vital chance was being lost due to the atrophy of the WHO's programme. He had a persuasive voice and the support of vaccine leaders in France with whom studies had been performed in Africa to show that a two-dose schedule of Salk's inactivated vaccine would be sufficient to stop polio in Africa (Fig. 3.3).[44]

Meanwhile, the landscape of international health was changing under the influence of James "Jim" Grant, executive director of the United Nation's International Children's Emergency Fund (UNICEF). Grant, a lawyer and internationalist, had been deeply influenced by the work of his father, John Grant, the medical missionary who had pioneered the training of barefoot doctors in China and who had been the first Professor of Public Health at the Rockefeller-funded Peking Union Medical College. In his role at UNICEF, Jim Grant had pledged to reduce the suffering and increase the well-being of the world's children, but how was this to be achieved at a time when the developing world was experiencing an economic recession? For Grant, the answer lay in prevention along the lines of the low-cost, high-impact targeted interventions that Ken Warren had been advocating. Indeed, Grant admired Warren's work and his dedication to the simple question of how the fruits of the biomedical sciences could be used to work for the poor majority in the Third World.[45]

---

[42]K. S. Warren, "Protecting the World's Children: An Agenda for the 1990s." *The Lancet*, 19 March 1988, p. 659.

[43]"Vaccine" comes from the Latin word *vacca*, meaning cow because cowpox scabs were first used to immunise against smallpox.

[44]Bill Foege, personal communication.

[45]J. Grant, Address to the New York Academy of Sciences L.S. Frohlich Award Conference 'Putting Biomedical Knowledge to Use in the Third World', 18 October 1988, UNICEF, p. 1.

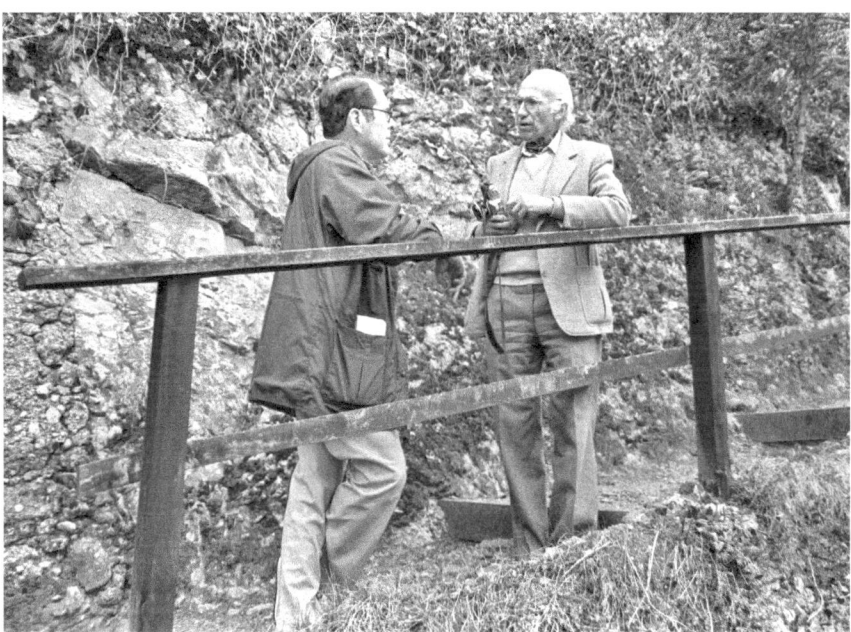

Fig. 3.3 Warren and Jonas Salk in conversation, Bellagio. Courtesy of Christopher Warren

Grant had become the executive director of UNICEF in 1980, and like Mahler at the WHO, as well as Warren, he was charismatic, idealistic, and determined to succeed. Through a combination of immutable moral force, providing funding for coordinated national programmes, and persuading political leaders to the cause, a global campaign to immunise the world's children was born in which Warren would play a substantial role. In 1983, Grant made the decisive move in terms of implementation with UNICEF's declaration of "A Children's Revolution." This was based on scientific and social advances that offered four vital new opportunities to improve the nutrition and health of the world's children: growth monitoring, oral-rehydration therapy, breast-feeding, and universal childhood immunisation.[46] "For all four actions the cost of the supplies and technology would be no more than a few dollars a day. Yet that could mean that literally hundreds of millions of young lives would be healthier. And within a decade, they could be saving the lives of 20,000 children each day. It is not the possibility of this kind of progress that is now in question, it is its priority."[47] Within months, Grant refined his focus still further by deciding to concentrate on UNICEF's initial efforts in the children's revolution solely on immunisation. The decision was salutary, guided as it was by the recent

---

[46]This policy became known by the acronym GOBI.

[47]K. S. Warren, "Tropical Medicine or Tropical Health: The Heath Clark Lectures", 1988, p. 152. Reviews of Infectious Diseases Vol. 12, No 1, January–February 1990. The University of Chicago Press.

eradication of smallpox, a landmark event in the history of medicine that was certified by the WHO in 1978, and the more contemporary success of the immunisation programme in the US. This US campaign to prevent the deaths of children from immunisable disease had been orchestrated by President Jimmy Carter. As soon as Carter entered the White House in January 1977, he invited his good friend Senator Dale Bumpers, Governor of Arkansas, and his wife Betty to Washington for dinner. Betty and the President's wife, Rosalynn, had been close friends when their husbands were governors. Both women were interested in public health, the plight of the poor in the southern states, and the role of immunisation in protecting the health of children. By the end of the dinner party, President Carter had been persuaded to the cause, and the following morning he telephoned Joseph Califarno, his Secretary of Health, Education, and Welfare asking what could be done to improve immunisation. Immediately Califarno telephoned the legendary Bill Foege, Head of the Centers for Disease Control and Prevention (CDC) in Atlanta. The Secretary of State asked Foege if it would be possible to set a goal of 90% of children being immunised before they started school. Foege takes up the story: "So, I asked my Director of Immunisation if 90% was feasible, and he said 'I would not want to see that in my job description,' so the next day we put it in his job description. And he rose to the occasion—soon we got 92%, then 93% and soon 95%. The interesting thing that we found was that the immunisation had to take place before school entry; if you really want to stop some of these diseases it had to be performed before the age of two."[48]

The differences between the US experience and the EPI was stark in terms of finance and strategy. In the US, ecumenical agencies came together: Carter and Califarno ensured that resources were in place, and the Public Health Service, the states, and the counties were united behind the programme. Importantly, a powerful coalition existed between the schools and parents. As Foege noted, "Once we decided to break measles transmission, that served as a tug-boat for the rest of immunisation."[49] Alas, no such cohesion existed for the global programme—It was starved of resources; surveillance was deficient; and country ministries of health lacked money and trained staff. Most debilitating of all was that a spirit of competition rather than cooperation existed between the WHO and UNICEF, and it would be some years before this relationship was transformed under the influence of the Task Force for Child Health.

These were the socio-medical forces that ushered Jonas Salk into Warren's office at the RF in May 1983. Although Warren had previously been skeptical about whether smallpox could be eradicated through vaccination, as June Goodfield writes in her authoritative social history of the immunisation story, "one of the most remarkable things about Ken was his capacity to change his mind."[50] Warren

[48]Bill Foege, personal communication.

[49]Bill Foege, personal communication.

[50]J. Goodfield, *A Chance to Live: The heroic story of the global campaign to immunise the world's children*. Macmillan, New York, 1991, p. 39.

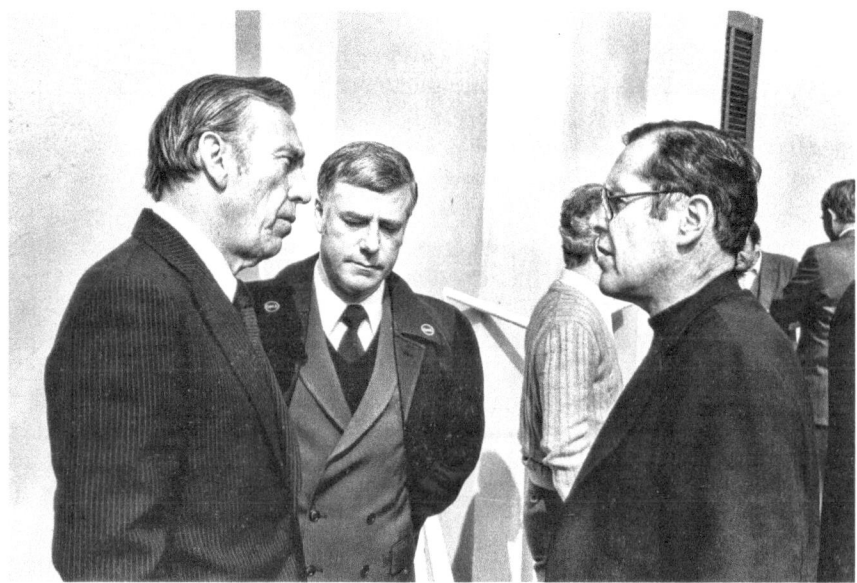

Fig. 3.4 Mahler and Warren, both men looking rather sombre, perhaps discussing their philosophical differences between WHO's 'Health for All by the Year 2000' and Selective Primary Heath Care. Standing in the *middle* of the photograph is the American medical researcher, Max Essex. Courtesy of Christopher Warren

immediately set himself the task of finding people with the skills, money, vision, and enthusiasm to support Grant, Salk, and others in making the children's revolution a reality. Before long, he had mobilised a cadre of experts to join him in the great humanitarian endeavour, including Robert McNamara of the World Bank, who he hoped would come up with the money. The one seemingly insurmountable obstacle to the aim of achieving universal childhood immunisation by 1990 was Halfdan Mahler and his implacable opposition to vertical campaigns. Warren, conscious of President Johnson's famous dictum concerning a tent and the position of J. Edgar Hoover, knew that it was only through a coordinated effort that the policy would stand any chance of success. After all, the WHO was the pre-eminent agency for health; it had the kudos, expertise, and organisational clout to spearhead the initiative. At the same time, Warren was determined to avoid any turf war developing between Mahler's WHO, Grant at UNICEF, and the RF, and he asked his friend Robert McNamara to fly to Geneva and persuade Mahler to join their campaign, which he duly did (Fig. 3.4).

All of the people involved in the preliminary discussions knew that the common enemy to the health of the poor remained poverty, but they also recognised that the immunisation programme offered the opportunity to launch one of the most audacious international health projects ever attempted—to protect the world's children from 6 killer diseases in 100 countries. It was agreed that a meeting should be organised to plan universal childhood immunisation at the Rockefeller

Foundation's Bellagio conference centre in Italy on March 12 to 16 1984, a gathering that would include the heads of WHO, UNICEF, the UN Development Programme (UNDP), the World Bank, and the Rockefeller Foundation as well as the directors of many of the major agencies dispensing bilateral aid such as the US Agency for International Development (USAID). Halfdan Mahler had agreed to attend the meeting, justifying his participation, according to Warren, "with the fact that the Expanded Programme on Immunisation was WHO's one vertical programme."[51] However, before the meeting in the Villa Serbelloni on Lake Como took place, there was a slightly bizarre turn of events involving Jim Grant, Halfdan Mahler, and Bill Foege. In the autumn of 1983, Mahler and Grant visited Foege at the CDC in Atlanta for what turned out to be an extraordinary conversation. Foege remembers that "there was just the two of them, and for a little while I believed that I was a therapist because they told me that 'we both have such big egos that we sometimes have trouble getting along' and you can imagine what it is like for WHO and UNICEF, because the same thing happens between organisations. But they said that they really wanted global immunisation to work, and that they did not want this kind of trouble between agencies. So their question was: is it possible to have an outside group that facilitates this but never co-ordinates it [the touted immunisation programme]? They did not want the word 'co-ordinate' to ever be used, because no big organisation wants to be co-ordinated. We eventually settled on the word 'facilitate', and they then suggested a Task Force outside any of the agencies to facilitate what they were doing. Then they asked me if the March 12–16, 1984 meeting at Bellagio ended up suggesting a Task Force, would I be willing to head it up? Then if so should it be in Geneva, New York or Washington DC? I told them that I would be willing to head up the Task Force, but that each of those places had a complication because it looks like you're favouring someone, so why not leave it in Atlanta and I wouldn't have to move (Fig. 3.5)."[52]

It would be difficult to imagine a more tranquil location for mediation than the Bellagio centre. In the past, Warren had used it as a place to identify and hammer out solutions to other enduring problems of public health, not least the preliminary discussions that had resulted in the Selective Primary Healthcare concept. For the 1984 event, less than 50 people attended the first Bellagio meeting. In addition to the main players, among others were D.A. Henderson, who had established the "ring of immunity" concept with the smallpox campaign; Gus Nossal; A.W. Causen, president of the World Bank; Ruhukana Rugunda, the Ugandan Minister of Health; and representatives from many health agencies in the developed world. The Bellagio meeting was recognition that the prevention of infection was not only better than its cure but was also much cheaper. A valuable lesson had also been learned by the international health community from the successful smallpox campaign: Although the vaccine for smallpox had been around for more than 200 years,

---

[51]K. S. Warren, 'The Alma-Ata Declaration: *Health for All by the Year 2000? Britannica Book of the Year*, *Encyclopedia Britannica*, Inc., Chicago, 1990, p. 27.

[52]Bill Foege, personal communication.

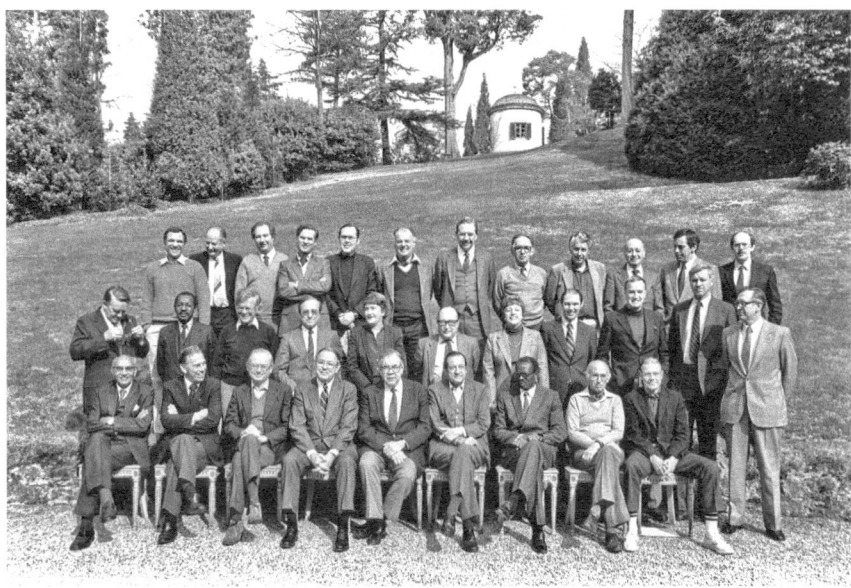

Fig. 3.5 Among the delegates to the first Bellagio conference in 1984 were: *left* to *right*, *top row* Ken Warren (5th), D.A. Henderson (7th), Gus Nossal (9th); *middle row* Ralph Henderson (8th), Bill Foege (10th); *bottom row* Halfdan Mahler (2nd), Jim Grant (6th), Jonas Salk (8th), and Robert McNamara (9th). Courtesy of Christopher Warren

it took little more than a decade for a coordinated campaign, adequately funded and brilliantly led, to achieve eradication.[53] The momentous decision to immunise all of the world's children was arrived at through a miasma of scepticism concerning both the strategy itself and the likelihood of achieving the objectives. Dr. Ruganda raised the central question of the conference: "Can it be performed? (Figs. 3.6 and 3.7)".[54]

The process of slow accretion set in motion by the EPI in 1974 was about to gather pace, yet even at Bellagio the depth of the moral, financial and ethical considerations weighed heavily on those involved. Gus Nossal, an expert in biotechnology and new vaccine research, witnessed some of the machinations unfold: "One of my favourite images of the meeting in Bellagio is a huffed up Mahler, the inspirational but not very effective director general of the WHO, Robert McNamara, and Jim Grant walking round and round and round the beautiful grounds of Bellagio with its steep side coming down from the villa to the sea, all of

---

[53]G. Nossal, "Protecting our Progeny: The Future of Vaccines." Perspective in Health Magazine, Special Centennial Edition, Vol. 7, No. 1, 2002.
[54]K. S. Warren, "Protecting the World's Children: An Agenda for the 1990s." *The Lancet*, 19 March 1988, p. 659.

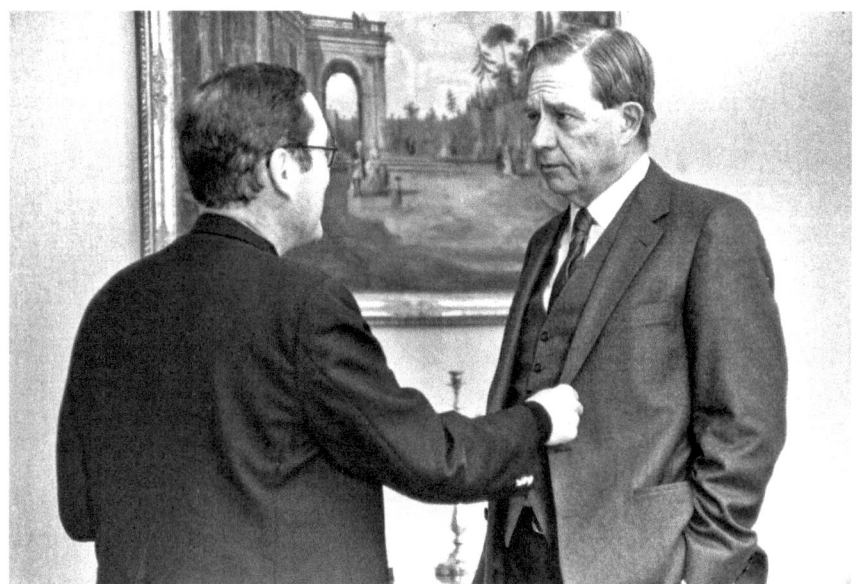

Fig. 3.6 A renowned advocate of moral force, here Warren amusingly uses some gentle physical force to get his point across to D.A. Henderson. Courtesy of Christopher Warren

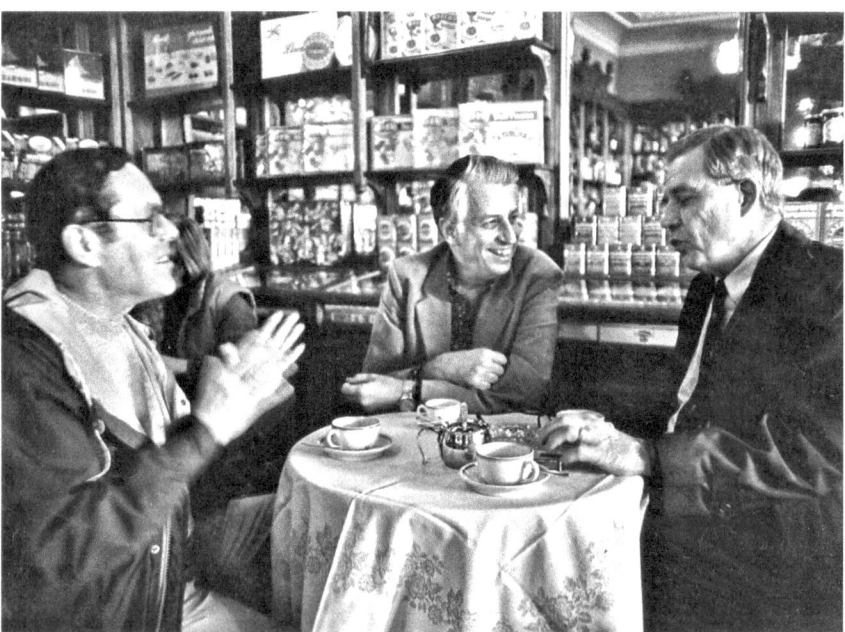

Fig. 3.7 Ken Warren, Gus Nossal (*centre*) and D.A. Henderson have coffee together in a local café on the banks of Lake Como, Italy. Courtesy of Christopher Warren

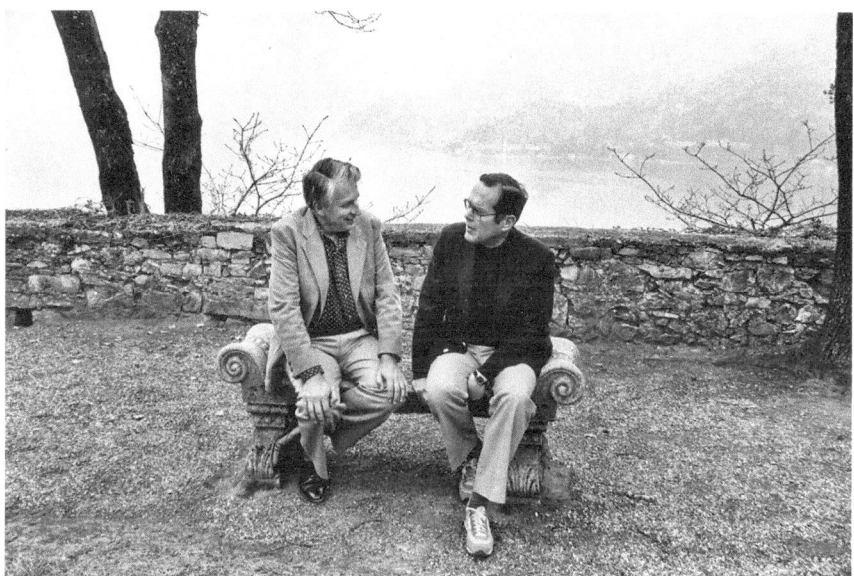

Fig. 3.8 Gus Nossal and Ken Warren deep in conversation, sitting on a bench in the grounds of the Villa Serbelloni, during a break from negotiations over the child immunisation programme. The immunologist, Gus Nossal, played an influential role in both Warren's GND network and the WHO's special programme for Research and Training in Tropical Diseases (TDR). Courtesy of Christopher Warren

them deep in conversation, deep in thought. And really that was the birth of the immunisation programme (Figs. 3.8 and 3.9)."[55]

Much to the relief of Grant and Mahler, at the close of the Bellagio meeting it was agreed that a Task Force for Child Survival would be formed to "facilitate" both country programmes and research aspects of accelerated immunisation activities with Bill Foege as Director. Foege was responsible to a group consisting of the five convening agencies: WHO, UNICEF, the World Bank, UNDP, and the Rockefeller Foundation. The Task Force met every 3 months for the next 5 years bringing together figures from the five organisations and other agencies to plan strategies and synchronise efforts. Only Warren and Ralph Henderson, director of the EPI, never missed a meeting.[56] Warren himself used the force of his personality to help keep the programme on track. Although he was a great proselytiser for the immunisation programme, his behaviour at the meetings struck an intriguing chord as recalled by Foege: "He [Warren] played a very interesting role in these quarterly meeting, because he was always so enthusiastic that early on in the meeting, he

---

[55]Gus Nossal, personal communication.

[56]Bill Foege, personal communication.

   J. Goodfield, *A Chance to Live*: *The heroic story of the global campaign to immunise the world's children*. Macmillan, New York, 1991, p. 51.

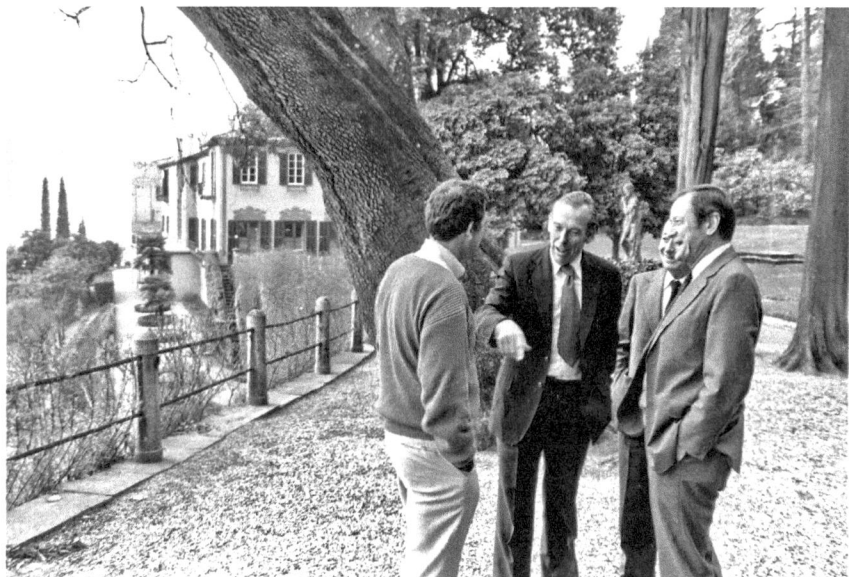

Fig. 3.9 Mahler facing the camera and Jim Grant (profiled in suit) in conversation in the grounds of the Villa Serbelloni, Bellagio. Courtesy of Christopher Warren

would say something that everyone objected to. People would just get angry and start talking back, and Ken was very easy in accepting the criticism, and pretty soon everyone would settle down, and we would get further than if we had never had that blow up… And I never knew whether Ken did this on purpose or whether it was just his enthusiasm and he wanted everyone to know what he was thinking at that moment. But it sure had an interesting effect on the group."[57] Conceivably, Warren was playing the role of devil's advocate, aiming to create a productive consensus, even to the detriment of himself. This was not a role that either his admirers or detractors had seen him adopt before, but if his emotional outbursts contributed to the success of the Task Force, he would have been inwardly contented (Figs. 3.10 and 3.11).

As ever, a major obstacle to the programme was money. Robert McNamara's speculation that the amount required to undertake the global campaign would be $100 million disheartened many. But although McNamara vouchsafed that he would raise the money, it was a young member of his staff, Amie Batson, who energised the mobilisation of the funds. She was prescient and talked of needing to raise billions rather than millions of dollars, and it was not until the AIDS pandemic that people came to understand that vast sums could be raised if the cause was important enough. For his part, Warren used his considerable network of contacts

---

[57]Bill Foege, personal communication.

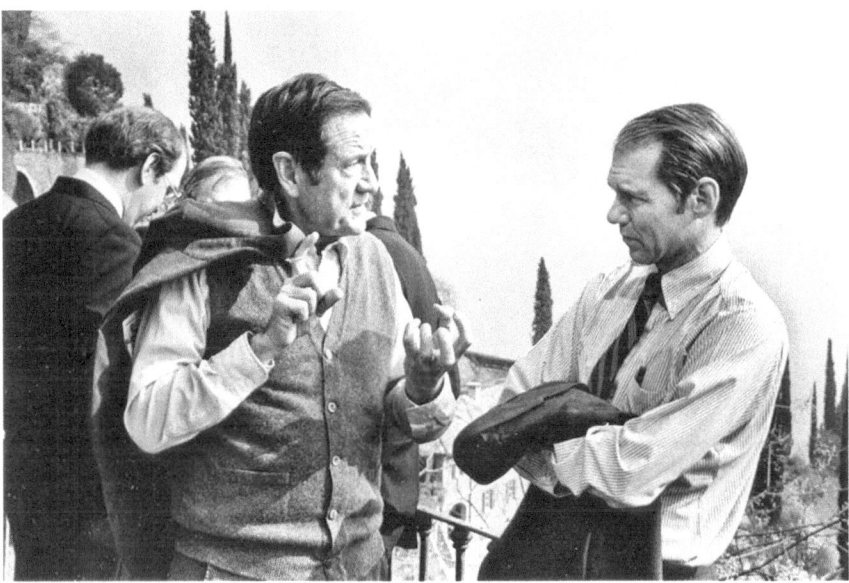

Fig. 3.10 On a balmy spring day at the first Bellagio conference, Jim Grant (*left*), Head of UNICEF, in conversation with Ralph (pronounced Rafe) Henderson, then of WHO. Courtesy of Christopher Warren

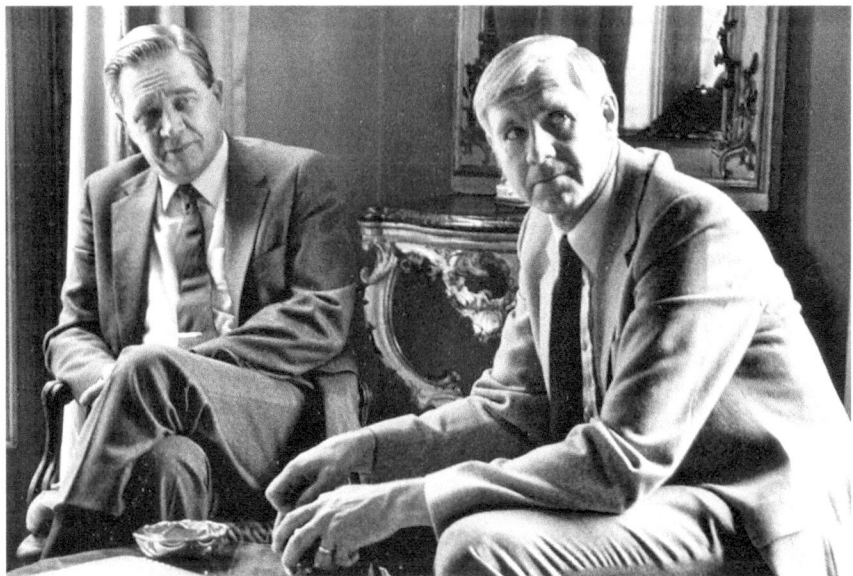

Fig. 3.11 On the *left* is D.A. Henderson, credited with leading smallpox eradication at WHO, Dean of Johns Hopkins School of Public Health. On the *right*, Bill Foege, Head of Task Force for Child Survival and lead negotiator between WHO and UNICEF. Courtesy of Christopher Warren

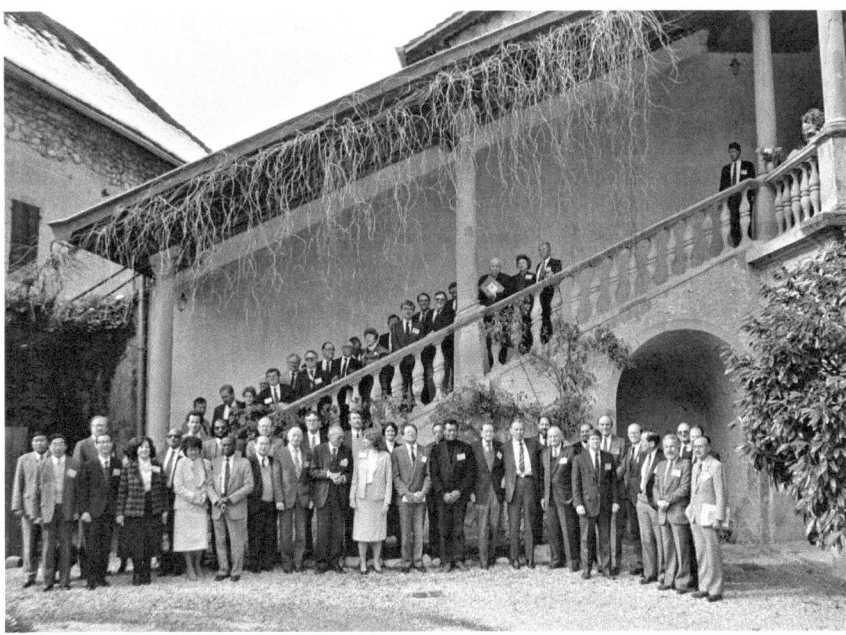

Fig. 3.12 Photograph of the delegates attending the Bellagio III in Talloires, France, 1988. Courtesy of Christopher Warren

and convening power to attract funding for the programme. A major contribution to the heightening of awareness was a 2-day meeting designed and organised by Warren at Rockefeller University especially for grant-makers, scientists, and the health-philanthropy community to advance the cause of child health. During the conference, Warren told the assembled delegates of the fun and gratification that came from a life in biomedical science and that "relatively small grants to laboratory research in the western world can greatly affect the development of new and more powerful vaccines."[58] In his capacity at the RF as a grant-maker, Warren also had a celebrated reputation in geographical medicine as a mobiliser of money. So memorable and persuasive was his performance at the conference that untapped reservoirs of patronage began to appear. Rebecca Rimel, for instance, joined the Pew Charitable Trusts, and then the Pew Memorial Trust, in 1983 as its Health Programme Manager and aimed to change the organisation's deliberately anonymous charitable profile in a purposeful manner. Today, she is the President and Chief Executive Officer at the Pew and is one of the most influential and experienced leaders of American philanthropy. Her rise to power began with feelings of trepidation when she made a telephone call to Warren in 1984: "Looking back,

---

[58]K. S. Warren, "In The New Age of Vaccines: U.S. Roles in an International Context." The Rockefeller University, New York, 22–23 October 1984, p. 4. Courtesy of the Pew Foundation archive.

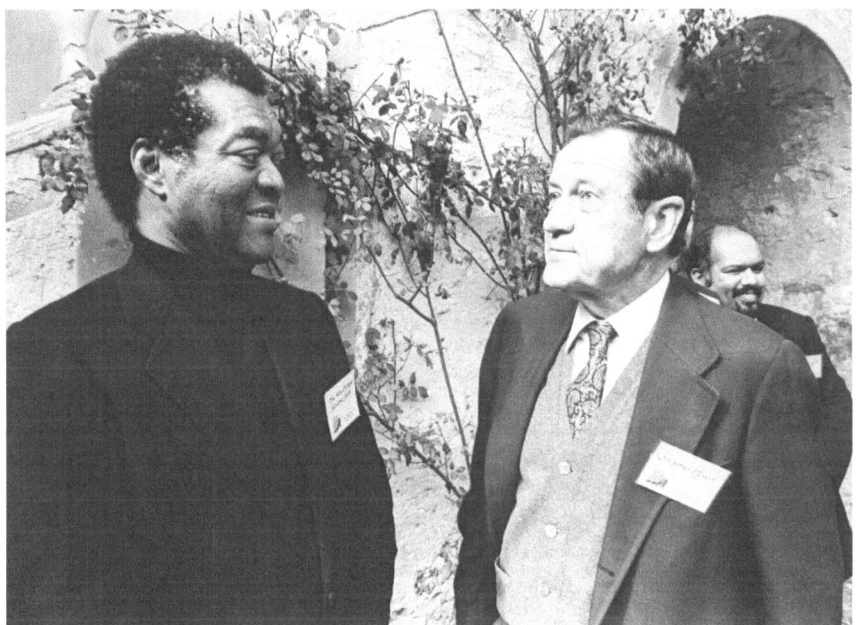

Fig. 3.13 Jim Grant and Olikoye Ransome Kuti, Minister of Health, Nigeria. Taken in Talloires, France in 1988 at 'Bellagio III' (March 10–12). The Declaration of Talloires was entitled, "Protecting the World's Children—An Agenda for the 1990s". Courtesy of Christopher Warren

I was incredibly naïve but I decided that we needed to do something, so I rang the Director of Health Sciences at the Rockefeller Foundation! I told him that we were small but that I wanted to make a difference and that we had funds to invest. After a moment, Ken said, 'How much have you got?' I said $3 million. His reply was 'Come over tomorrow!' This led to our work on epidemiology and antibiotic resistance research that we are doing today. Ken could be scary and dismissive if he thought that you weren't serious and he didn't suffer fools. I owe him so much. He took a risk with us, but it turned out very well."[59]

Alongside gaining much-needed funding for the global vaccination campaign, so began the career of a new actor in the international health field and a coordinated campaign with the RF and the WHO in vaccine development that sought to exploit biotechnology to produce vaccines for hepatitis A, respiratory viruses, dengue fever, meningitis, and tuberculosis. Warren had his finger on the pulse of American philanthropy; he was determined to raise funds for new vaccines to address the three greatest killers of children: diarrheal diseases, respiratory diseases, and malaria. Warren was unequivocal; he believed that the RF shared a responsibility for diseases anywhere on the globe (Figs. 3.12, 3.13, 3.14 and 3.15).

---

[59]Rebecca Rimel, personal communication.

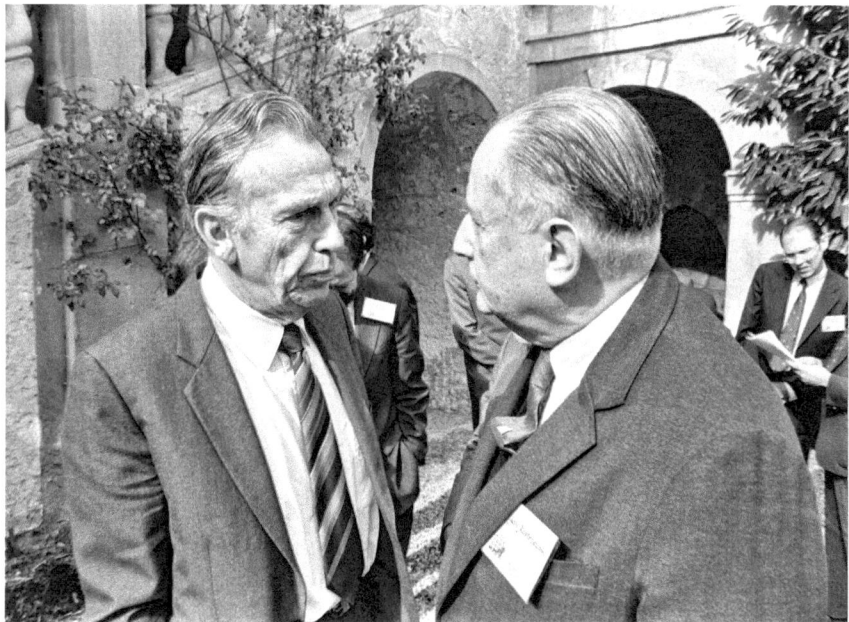

Fig. 3.14 Mahler in conversation with the epidemiologist, Professor Jan Kostrzewski, Talloires, France, 1988. Courtesy of Christopher Warren

Warren remained a pivotal figure in the series of three eponymous Bellagio meetings, with the original 1984 conference being referred to as "Bellagio I," "Bellagio II" held in Colombia in 1985, and "Bellagio III" held in March 1988 at Talloires, France. During that period, a transformation took place: universal childhood immunisation levels reached almost 80% by 1990. Immediately after the Bellagio meeting, several countries took the initiative to immunise all of their children. President Belisario Belancur of Columbia led a massive national effort by mobilizing all segments of society—from priests in the confessional to Boy Scouts and the Army—to immunise the children of his country. In 1985, when Bellagio II was held in Cartagena, Columbia, 90 world leaders and public health experts were in attendance. Not only was remarkable progress reported in several countries, but the world's two most populous nations, India and China, wholeheartedly joined the effort. UNICEF's *State of the World's Children* report for 1983 had estimated that 5 million unimmunised children were dying each year, but through immunisation that number had been reduced to 3.5 million. Obviously the planned miracle had fallen short, but for the 1.5 million children who would otherwise have died prematurely, the long scientific journey from Edward Jenner to Bellagio had been life-enhancing. In 1960, 1 in 3 children died in the first year of life; in 1988, the figure was 1 in 4. To celebrate this health outcome metamorphosis, Grant, Mahler, Foege, and Warren completed "The Declaration of Talloires," a document that examined how momentum could be sustained and what other effective measures

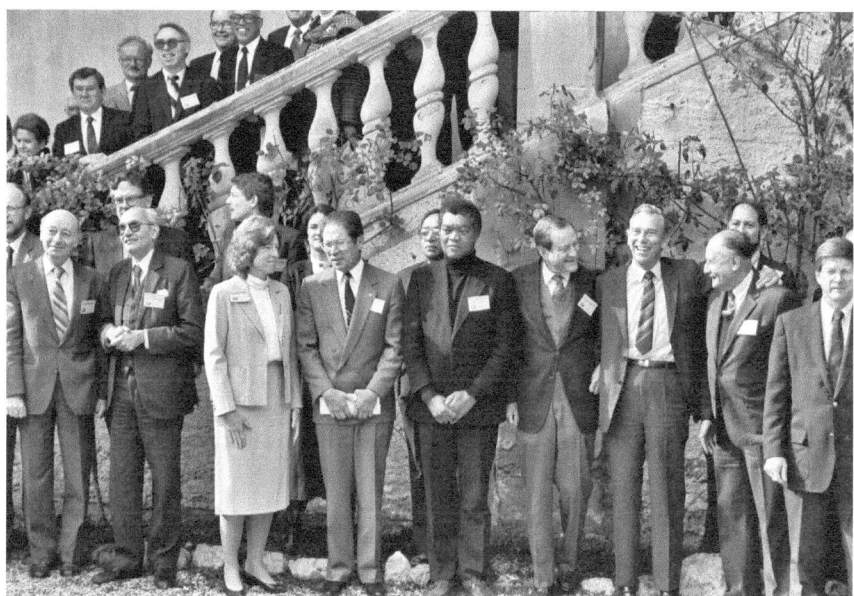

Fig. 3.15 Olikoye Ransome-Kuti, centre, on his *left* Jim Grant, and then Mahler. At the *right* edge of photograph, in spectacles, is Kenneth Prewitt of the Rockefeller Foundation. Courtesy of Christopher Warren

could be added. This declaration had resonance with the Declaration of Alma-Ata, which enshrined health as "a fundamental human right." But how times had changed. By 1988, the alliance was dissolving, and different problems demanded attention. Warren was about to leave the RF after more than a decade of service, whereas Mahler would relinquish his post at the WHO to become secretary-general of the International Planned Parenthood Federation in 1989. Ten years earlier, the men represented two philosophically different approaches to addressing the health of the world's poorest people; however, where once there had been distrust, now there was empathy. A scene at Talloires captures how those macro-differences were played out at a micro-level as Mahler realised that the great venture was coming to an end. Throwing an arm around Ken Warren's shoulder, Mahler was heard to say, "Look, my friend, you and I will never retire. We'll go on being subversive terrorists for health forever."[60]

---

[60]J. Goodfield, *A Chance to Live: The heroic story of the global campaign to immunise the world's children.* Macmillan, New York, 1991, p. 170.

Chapter 4
Boundaries, Frontiers, and Disciplines

Warren, according to Adel Mahmoud, "had limitless energy" and as a consequence was restless if he wasn't working. In parallel to his achievements in child immunisation, Warren continued his "subversive" work across a wide spectrum of health-related subjects. These diverse projects reflected his personal character: his love of literature, his championing of technology, and his ability to cross traditional disciplinary boundaries.

As the GND programme was being launched, another idea began to germinate in Warren's mind, which he hoped would contribute to the accumulated knowledge of parasitic diseases: training people from the developing world in modern scientific techniques with the objective of developing therapies against parasitic infections. His vision was to emulate the spectacular development of molecular biology orchestrated by a seminar course at Cold Spring Harbor Laboratory given by the Phage group. To achieve this aim, he formed an advisory committee, which included Joshua Lederberg, President of the Rockefeller Foundation; James Henry, President of the Edna McConnell Clark Foundation; and Richard Krause, Director of the National Institute of Allergy and Infectious Diseases. At the first meeting of the committee in January 1979, Lederberg suggested that the time was ripe for a similar course in parasitology.[1] The group's initial attempt to establish a summer course in the biology of parasitism was rebuffed by the governing body of Cold Spring Harbor, but they were welcomed with open arms by Paul Gross, Director of the Marine Biological Laboratory in Woods Hole, Massachusetts. He was enthusiastic about creating a course that would combine parasitology with state-of-the-art science.

Reminiscent of a biological organism itself, the Marine Biological Laboratory (MBL) had evolved from its late 19th century origins to become a crossroads of scientific ideas that was a beating heart of developmental progress. Its geographical setting, combined with the allure of discovery, fascinated physician–writers and

---

[1]K. S. Warren & C. C. Jimenez (eds), *The Great Neglected Diseases of Mankind Biomedical Research Network: 1978–1988*. New York: The Rockefeller Foundation, 1988, p. 329.

© Springer International Publishing AG 2017
C. Keating, *Kenneth Warren and the Great Neglected Diseases of Mankind Programme*, Springer Biographies,
DOI 10.1007/978-3-319-50147-5_4

attracted academics down from Boston and students from around the world. Gerald Weissmann, in his book, *The Woods Hole Cantata*, captures the aquatic adhesion felt by generations of natural scientists to the area's distinct geography: "For nearly a hundred summers, biologists have gathered near the deep channel that joins Vineyards Sound to Buzzards Bay at Woods Hole. Most of these scholars have at one time or other performed the classic experiment of the Marine Biological Laboratory: They have fertilised urchin eggs with urchin sperm in a small dish. Sea urchins, or, to give them their formal name in Massachusetts, *Arbacia punctulata*, are ubiquitous in these waters; their fertile season happily overlaps the long vacation of academic calendars."[2]

When Warren travelled to Woods Hole in 1979 to meet with Paul Gross, he was accompanied by Josh Lederberg, Anthony Cerami, and Joe Cook, the latter of the Edna McConnell Clark Foundation. The men hoped that collectively that they would be able to fund the parasitology course if Gross's institution could host the endeavour. Warren attracted many epithets during his career, some endearing ("inherently charismatic"), others less so ("egotistic jerk"), but one that fitted unambiguously during his years at the RF was "philanthropoid." The term was first used by Dewin R. Embree, who served as secretary of the RF in the early 1920s. According to Embree, a philanthropoid was someone who makes a living by giving away other people's money.[3] It was to this group of philanthropids at the RF that Warren belonged as he continued the quest to design a formula for financing the new breed of scientists who would advance human well-being. Because of their almost constant travel throughout the international scientific community, the early Rockefeller philanthropoids became known as "circuit riders."[4] Warren was the archetypal circuit rider, and he hoped that Joe Cook's participation in the project would bring added scientific gravitas alongside that additional prerequisite, finance.

Joe Cook immediately saw the long-term value of bringing students from the developing world to Woods Hole and training them over a period of 10 weeks to provide sufficient practical contact with the techniques of molecular and cell biology to enable the students to feel comfortable about applying such methods on their return home. As Joe recalled, "Ken made all these contacts, and he suggested that one thing that would help parasitology was this course. Anyway, at the meeting with Paul Gross, it was accepted that the RF and the Edna McConnell Clark Foundation (EMCF) would provide the funds. I'm not sure whether this may have been [another] case of making horse and rabbit stew with EMCF providing the horse and Ken the rabbit, but I believe it was, and continues to be, a good stew … It

---

[2]G. Weissmann, *The Woods Hole Cantata, Essays on Science and Society*. New York, 1985, p. 109.

[3]G. Jonas, *The Circuit Riders: Rockefeller Money and the Rise of Modern Science*. W.W. Horton & Company, New York and London, 1989, p. 63.

[4]The term 'circuit riders' refers to the early disciples of John Wesley, who travelled ceaselessly on horseback to bring the word of God to out-of-the-way places.

was an important course, and very important for bringing people into parasitology research."[5]

Warren ensured the success of the endeavour by persuading the immunologist John David to become the first Director of the Biology of Parasitism Course, a position that he held with distinction, and which convinced David, an "innocent immunologist," to explore "the tangled fields of immunoparasitology."[6] At a conference in New Orleans in October 1980, dedicated to *The Current Status and Future of Parasitology* jointly sponsored by the RF and the Josiah Marry Jr. Foundation, Paul Gross described the development of the course: "The problem was to convince the MBL Corporation and trustees that some of their already limited resources should be pre-empted for a major new educational programme in parasitology... Beyond convincing one's colleagues that something ought to be done, there were other problems: acquiring a physical plant suitable for the highly sophisticated teaching we were considering; providing an adequate small mammal facility; and ensuring biosafety control regardless of our own views about the reality of perceived hazards."[7] Well might the director of the MBL have underscored these apprehensions, as when John David arrived at Woods Hole in the summer of 1979, combined with a palpable sense of discovery, there was some understandable trepidation about standards of health and safety. David recalls how their course formed a break with the Woods Hole tradition: "Remember we had nothing to do with marine biology, there was not a single marine parasite—this was human parasites. They [Corporation and the trustees] were very scared about the animals, so we had animal rooms that were like [secure] agricultural departments with double doors ... because they were worried about parasites escaping."[8] The main object of the course was to bring together the new concepts and tools of immunology, molecular biology, and membrane biochemistry to the problems of parasitology. A further aim was to attract scientists to this area. The latter goal was accomplished through a combination of digging through Warren's capacious scientific Rolodex—he prided himself on his connections—and the integrity of the ideal. Recruitment moved ahead rapidly as directed by Warren, David, and the Harvard parasitologist and medical historian, Eli Chernin.

The course was an immediate success, but it got off to an unconventional start when the NIH malariologist Louie Miller brought chickens with malaria—*Plasmodium gallinaceum*—to Woods Hole in his car! This alarmed even the normally unflappable John David, who remembers being "scared stiff that this could lead to all the sea gulls in Woods Hole dying of malaria." All went well, however,

---

[5]Joe Cook, personal communication.

[6]J. David in K. S. Warren & C. C. Jimenez (eds), *The Great Neglected Diseases of Mankind Biomedical Research Network: 1978–1988*. New York: The Rockefeller Foundation, 1988, p. 15.

[7]P. R. Gross, "Appendix III: The biology of Parasitism Course at the Marine Biological Laboratory Woods Hole Massachusetts," in K. S. Warren & C. C. Jimenez (eds), *The Great Neglected Diseases of Mankind Biomedical Research Network: 1978–1988*. New York: The Rockefeller Foundation, 1988, p. 329.

[8]John David, personal communication.

and the course didn't disturb the ecological system or the intellectual tranquility of the MBL.[9] David's tenure as director lasted 5 years, and the summer of 1979 set a pattern for the immense influence of the course, which still continues today. There was little free time because the laboratory work was demanding; yet, on weekends and in the long hot mid-summer evenings, excitement filled the air because there was a shared belief that if questions about parasitology needed to be asked, this was the best place in the world to ask them. The children of the participants were not forgotten: Special educational classes were offered throughout the summer vacation. A nascent sense of camaraderie grew when the parasitologists became the volleyball champions of the MBL, and new multicultural friendships were formed over picnics at the local beach, a small strip of sand "hardly big enough for a committee, but close enough to the laboratories so that the investigators can walk down for a sandwich lunch with their children on sunny weekends."[10] Approaching the shoreline, the sounds of beach life could be heard before the crowd came into view, particularly if Ken Warren had a microphone, rhapsodizing the gathering for being the most fantastic group of people in the world and how their work was going to fundamentally change the world for the better.[11] No one was in any doubt: Of crucial importance to the Woods Hole course was to have some fun along the way.

Warren's desire to get people involved in parasitology was insatiable, although the serious side of science was leavened by an equal determination to create a light-touch atmosphere of collegiate good humor and enjoyment. One of the first jobs that Warren asked John Bruer to do in his role as a visiting research fellow at the RF was to organise the inaugural course at Woods Hole. Having had some unfortunate experiences with biomedical scientists in the past, Bruer's first emotion on arriving at Woods Hole was one of apprehension, however, any unease was soon displaced by enjoyment: "When I got there we would sit around and have drinks and conversations with John David, Gus Nossal, Tony Cerami and listen to Phil Marsden speaking about his life studying the natural history of tropical diseases and being the Medical Officer for all of North Africa... I've got to say, it was a lot of fun."[12] The Woods Hole natives were friendly, too: Debbie and Al Senft's clam bakes were legendary, and they offered an open invitation to their home to the members of the course. Debbie Senft is the granddaughter of Frederick T. Gates, the American Baptist minister who was the principal philanthropic adviser to John D. Rockefeller.[13] Sylvia Warren also remembers lobster picnics taking place on the beach, the feelings of excitement, fun, and of people entertaining one another in the

[9]John David, personal communication.

[10]L. Thomas, *The Lives of a Cell: Notes of a Biology Watcher*, The Viking Press, 1974, p. 61.

[11]Dick Guerrant, personal communication.

[12]John Bruer, personal communication.

[13]Frederick T. Gates, credited with urging the idea of the RF on John D. Rockefeller, said to his fellow trustees in his last meeting as a member of the board, "When you die and come to approach the judgement of Almighty God, what do you think He will demand of you? Do you for an instant presume to believe that He will inquire into your petty failures or your trivial virtues? No! He will ask just one question: 'What did you do as a trustee of the Rockefeller Foundation?'".

beautiful marine setting.[14] The resulting intellectual fireworks and exchanges of ideas between the young investigators from across the world formed a welcome counterbalance to the hard lonely work, and near persistent failures, associated with science. The laboratory experiments, the talk, the interchange, and the people formed the dynamic ingredients of success, thus bringing a new generation into the field with more laboratories devoted to parasitic diseases. Warren was a magnet for what was best in research by recognizing that it was only through research that the complex problems of parasitic disease could be solved.

The first 10-week course was limited to 16 students, and it still is today, with 50% coming from the developing world (including 3 from Kenya) where most of the parasitic diseases being studied were indigenous.[15] There was no formal application process, and according to John David, the intake was limited to 16 because that was the maximum number that the laboratory room could take. John takes up the story: "We were interested in getting about half the students from overseas, as many of these were excellent applicants and we tried to get everyone from graduate students, to fellows, to faculty to even professors. We got the WHO and the Wellcome to help fund some of the students. As I was going to Brazil regularly, we let the people in many of the big cities know about the programme, as did the first Brazilians who attended the programme. But we succeeded in attracting people from all over the world, including Africa, Asia, Europe and the Americas.[16] The researchers were there to learn about modern biology, biochemistry, immunology and molecular biology. This experience, according to Onesmo ole-MoiYoi, was to prove invaluable; his own scientific career had been redirected by Ken Warren, and he believes that when those students returned home, "they were completely transformed."[17] The 10-week course had an infectious influence on the students because their training gave them new tools to better understand their countries' indigenous diseases. During the first year's programme, the students produced monoclonal antibodies to *Leishmania enrietti* and showed that several of these reacted with tubulin. They isolated messenger RNA from malaria, tyrpanosomes, leishmania, and ameba and translated parasite polypeptides in vitro. They also followed the complete life cycle of Aedes aegypti mosquitoes, of malaria using *Plasmodium gallinaceum*, and of *Schistosoma mansoni*. What's more, the experience led many of the students to switch to parasitology, thus helping to bring a new generation of developing world scientists into the field (Fig. 4.1).

Rather than having a destabilizing influence on the institutional ecology of the MBL, the course added a layer of intellectual luster to its spirit of science, congeniality, and distinguished history. Even as early as 1980, Paul Gross believed vindicated by his decision to offer a home to the new course that combined parasitology with modern biomedical science: "Our conclusions about the course are in

---

[14]Sylvia Warren, personal communication.

[15]John David, personal communication.

[16]John David, personal communication.

[17]Onesomo ole-MoiYoi, personal communication.

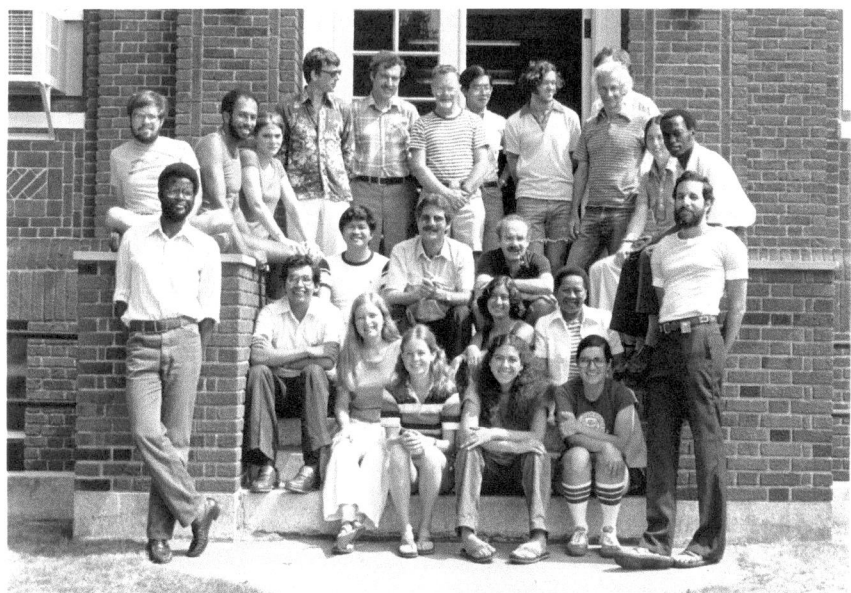

Fig. 4.1 The inaugural biology of parasitism class, Woods Hole, 1980. Courtesy of The Marine
Biological Laboratory Archives

a report we sent to Cook and Warren, whose aid, and that of the two great foundations they represent, was critical to the entire undertaking. In summary, I wrote
that I have participated in, or observed the first offering of, many advanced courses,
sometimes in the guise of a teacher, sometimes as a department chairman, and
recently as a dean. None of these offerings was as complex, as specialised, nor as
original an undertaking as the MBL 'Biology of Parasitism' course. None was so
quickly brought to effective and predictable function. Everyone associated with the
effort, not the least among them the foundation's staff and the MBL support staff,
deserved the thanks of the biological community."[18]

The Woods Hole course was part of Warren's synchronised plan for the initial
reduction and eventual elimination of parasitic diseases that exact such a high cost
in human suffering and economic loss. It evolved in tandem with his GND network,
which funded parasite-drug development with Yongyuth Yuthavong's group at
Mahidol University in Thailand and Tony Cerami's team at Rockefeller University,
which performed groundbreaking research work in Kenya. Indeed, Warren's former
group at Case Western Reserve University went on to establish a strong presence in
field of malaria research in Africa and Papua New Guinea. Long-term planning and

---

[18]P. R. Gross, "Appendix III: The biology of Parasitism Course at the Marine Biological
Laboratory Woods Hole Massachusetts." in K. S. Warren & C. C. Jimenez (eds), *The Great
Neglected Diseases of Mankind Biomedical Research Network: 1978–1988*. New York: The
Rockefeller Foundation, 1988, p. 330.

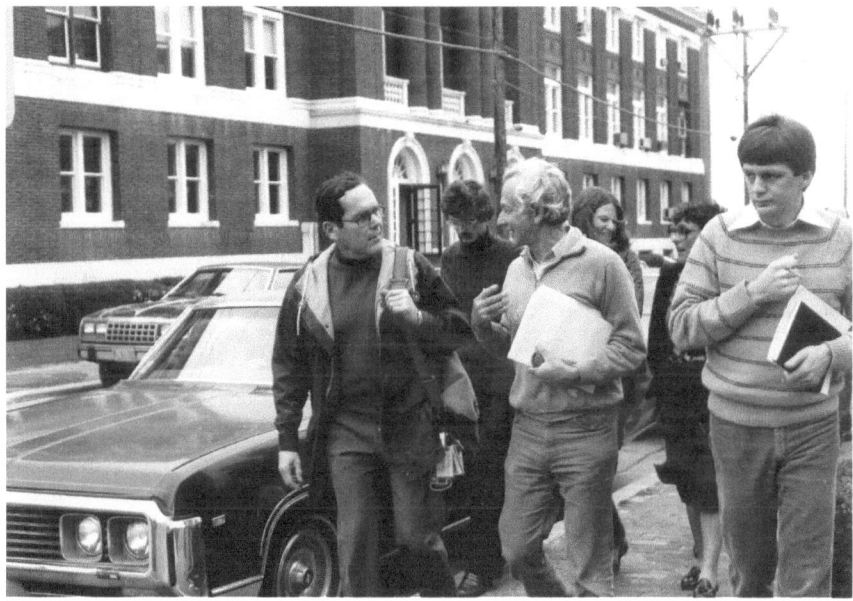

Fig. 4.2 Intellectual bustle in the air with Warren, John David and colleagues on their way to the Biology of Parasitism Course, Woods Hole. Courtesy of Christopher Warren

organisation on an international scale were strategies applied by Warren to guarantee that the future in parasitology would be productive.

In 1980, additional financial support was given by the Tropical Disease Research Programme of the WHO and by the Wellcome Trust, which was an acknowledgement of the course's material contributions to the field of parasitology. These accomplishments, brought about in 2 short years, more than justified the hopes of those who planned and supported the course at its inception. It led John David to write this summation of the fertile atmosphere that had been created at Woods Hole: "The intellectual excitement and enthusiasm generated by the interactions between faculty and students has led to a plethora of new ideas that have already had a fertilising influence in home institutions all over the world. This course has been directly responsible for new collaborations and new research that would not have existed without it, for a number of gifted new workers coming into the field, and for establishing a feeling of warm and generous communication and exchange of ideas (Fig. 4.2)."[19]

For many, the Biology of Parasitism (BOP) course was a rite of passage, a magnet, and a mecca for those enthralled by biology that had a very special

[19]J. David in "Appendix III: The biology of Parasitism Course at the Marine Biological Laboratory Woods Hole Massachusetts," in K. S. Warren & C. C. Jimenez (eds), *The Great Neglected Diseases of Mankind Biomedical Research Network: 1978–1988*. New York: The Rockefeller Foundation, 1988, p. 334.

environment and which still remains today a premier course for parasitology. One scientist who has had an enduring relationship with the courses is Dyann Wirth, Co-Chair of the Infectious Disease Initiative, for not only was Wirth a member of the inaugural class, she also taught on the course. "I was in the class and there weren't any molecular biologists on the faculty, because there weren't really any molecular biologists. At the time, I was a postdoc at Harvard in Wally Gilbert's Laboratory and I was trained in molecular biology, so I ended up teaching the molecular biology part of the course for another four years. The BOP led me to getting a job in parasitology, so it was a huge influence on my career."[20] Moreover, together with her colleagues, Lex Van der Ploegh and Jeffrey Ravetch, Wirth established the highly influential Molecular Parasitology Autumn meetings which became a successful forum for graduate students and postdocs to rub shoulders with leading figures in the field and to have their abstracts selected for a talk at Woods Hole. Some of the former students that went on to become renowned researchers include Norma Andrews, Photini Sine, Ricardo Gazzinelli, and James "Jay" Bangs.

For proximal as well as historical reasons, the BOP course continues to retain a magical quality and is inextricably associated with the Woods Hole community not merely as seasonal scientific interlopers but as a constant leitmotif of its history and culture. Independence Day celebrations in Woods Hole bear witness to an out-pouring of patriotic fervor—original flags with 13 stars can be seen, a classic 1966 Ford Bronco might slowly pass as a carnival atmosphere beings to build. All sections of the community join together on July 4th, and since 1980, the BOP students and faculty have been making their own idiosyncratic contribution. Original, flamboyant visceral and scientifically outrageous—no one forgets the BOP contribution to the annual procession! Various helminth infections of humans —including nematodes, trematodes, and cestodes—have been constructed and presented to the good people of Woods Hole. In 2016, the celebrated American scientist and former GND Career Development Fellow, Alan Sher, who in the past had impersonated a malaria-infected red blood cell and a worm, was seen encased in a deep brown muslin sheet secured by a bright red four inch–wide ribbon. The mummified immunobiologist, who had come as a "bloody stool," was accompanied by colleagues and students, some of whom were masquerading as a giant amoeba! After watching the evening fireworks display, which took place in Falmouth Harbor, the BOP "family" ended the day huddled around tables discussing science while drinking beer in the back room of their favorite bar, The Captain Kidd. For those fortunate people who found the time to walk on the beach at Buzzard's Bay at sunset and experience the bioluminescent ctenophores, the memory will never fade.[21]

---

[20]Dyann Wirth, personal communication.

[21]Tom Coleman, personal communication.

INCLEN

Although the concept of what constitutes neglected tropical diseases is very much at the forefront of the global health debate today, the other central policy of the RF's Health Sciences Division, the International Clinical Epidemiology Network (INCLEN), has become increasingly anonymous in the history of geographical medicine. INCLEN was the brainchild of the urbane Canadian epidemiologist, Kerr White, a physician who built a distinguished career expounding the essential role of primary care in any well-balanced health care system and who was Warren's deputy at the RF. For White, primary care was of crucial importance when considering the needs of the entire population. White's approach to health had been shaped by a year-long visit to England in the late 1950s, where he immersed himself in the science of epidemiology, coming under the influence of the discipline's intellectual giants: Bradford Hill, Donald Reid, Jerry Morris, Archie Cochrane, and Richard Doll.[22] He assimilated their ideas, i.e., the connection between social conditions and disease, the theory of randomisation, the need for evidence-based medicine, and the power of medical statistics.

White was implacably opposed to the view that there was only one approach to understanding diseases, a belief that he believed arose from the separation of schools of public health from medical schools. Furthermore, he pointed the finger of blame at the Rockefeller Foundation's well-meaning officers in 1918 who had financially annexed population-focused approaches from clinical and the laboratory perspectives. These three approaches became separated, and White famously used Johns Hopkins as the example of how this well-intentioned idea had unforeseen consequences. He observed that there were two institutions in Baltimore: Johns Hopkins Medical School and the School of Public Health, both separated by Wolfe Street. If someone were to put a layer of dust on Wolfe Street, he suggested, there would be no footprints between the two august institutions.[23] In other words, there existed an invisible Berlin Wall that caused an ideological divide. According to White, this resulted in those investigators familiar with the population perspective being separated intellectually and culturally from the biomedical investigators and teachers who were making extraordinary advances in the understanding of disease processes. The latter, however, were contributing much less to the understanding of the multiple social, behavioural, psychological, environmental, occupational, and nutritional factors that influence both health and disease. Clinical epidemiology was funded specifically to bridge the gap by (1) co-opting medical people, (2) awakening their interest, (3) showing them the continuity between the health conditions their patients experienced and the diseases with which they presented, and (4) making it clear that if they wanted to be real doctors, they should concern themselves with these related issues.

---

[22]C. Keating, *Smoking Kills: The Revolutionary Life of Richard Doll*. Oxford: Signal Books, 2009.
[23]Scott Halstead, personal communication.

Intriguingly, John Knowles, president of the RF, interviewed Kerr White for the position of Director of Health Sciences before eventually appointing Warren to the role. During the 1970s, White and Knowles had numerous discussions about the growing divide between medicine and public health and what might be done to improve the impasse. Knowles knew that in Warren he had a director with vision and tropical health experience who would deliver the GND programme, and in 1979, he appointed Kerr White as Deputy Director of the Health Sciences Division. White was 12 years older than Warren, and their demeanour, management styles, and approaches were poles apart, as John Bruer remembers: "Kerr White was a very different character from Ken, about 180 degrees opposed. He was a Canadian, but very *British*; a dignified quiet man. Ken was always exceedingly enthusiastic about things, wanted things done yesterday—but overall a fun guy to be around, inspiring. But I remember one time in particular being in an elevator with Ken and Kerr, and Ken was going on about something that 'had to be done, it had to be done!' Kerr and I just looked at each other and thought 'what the hell is going on…?' He was a nice counterpoise to Ken."[24] White's appointment was welcomed by Warren because he admired his colleague's abilities and had got to know him when he was a Trustee of Case Western Reserve University. Perhaps what was less welcomed was the allocation of approximately half the budget of the Division of Health Sciences to get INCLEN started.

Despite their differing personal styles, Warren and White loved their work and were conscious of their roles as custodians of the RF's enormous accomplishments in the field of health. Both were beneficiaries of Knowles' science-based development programme, nurtured under his presidency, of which INCLEN was a huge new project with the aim of creating hundreds of epidemiologists around the world. In 1979, Roy Acheson, the eminent British epidemiologist, helped to launch the INCLEN programme by organising its first seminar for clinicians at Churchill College, Cambridge. Writing in *The Lancet* in 2003, White believed that his friend's efforts helped to get INCLEN off to the excellent start that was critical to its success: "By assembling an international roster of distinguished academicians, including a Nobel Laureate, he [Acheson] seemed to have helped them to convince the gathering of young clinicians from medical schools in the developing world that a population's health was as worthy of investigation as biomedical processes."[25] INCLEN was dedicated to strengthening clinical epidemiology in the Third World through local training in these skills. It went on to establish an integrated system with five sites in the United States, Canada, and Australia that over the following decade trained more than 1400 young medical school faculty who went on to staff clinical research units in some 80 medical schools in 33 countries including sites in Africa, China, Europe, Latin America, and Southeast Asia. The objective was to teach physicians how to conduct research on their countries' most serious health problems in order to shape less-costly and more effective health policies.

---

[24]John Bruer, personal communication.
[25]*The Lancet*, Vol. 362, 19 July 2003, p. 253.

Historically, the philosophy that had guided the RF's philanthropy was to use its money to lead the way and for others to follow. The INCLEN project was therefore its ideal vehicle: The theory was one of "show what can be done, and then let others develop the work." Warren's work followed this principle on a grand scale. His main problem, however, was that if the programmes under his Health Sciences umbrella were to be truly long-lasting, they would need to attract new funding streams. This search for benefactions would prove to be a chronic source of frustration and disappointment, especially for the clinical epidemiology programme.

Kerr White left the RF in 1984, at the age of 67, having been kept on past the mandatory retirement age of 65. A year earlier, Warren's thoughts had already turned to finding a replacement deputy director, and he decided to contact his friend and fellow medical scientist, Scott Halstead. Halstead was working in the laboratory at Fort Detrick on sabbatical leave when he got a call from Ken asking, "How would you like to change your venue?" Halstead immediately said yes and showed up for work in October 1983.[26] Halstead was a physician of experience in the tropics, setting up the first laboratory to study dengue in Bangkok and later acting as a consultant for the WHO to the 10 countries in Asia where dengue was endemic. For the next few years, INCLEN prospered under the protective supervision of Halstead, a time when the annual meetings got bigger, better, and more fun. Halstead saw it as an altogether brilliant time for the RF with INCLEN and the GND being complimentary, built along similar lines, and pursuing goals by educating a younger generation. Some other international-health strategists disagreed, seeing an inherent dilemma between the GND, which used basic science to reduce the burden of disease, and INCLEN, which favoured clinical epidemiology.[27] However, for Halstead no such blurring of lines existed: "INCLEN was always directed at studies on interventions for patients and therefore not laboratory-based per se. There is no dichotomy between observations made in a clinical setting on human responses to disease or therapy, and basic science understanding of the physiology or pharmacy involved. Information gained from observations on humans can and does refer back to strengthen or contradict basic science understanding, and thus helps to frame new basic research questions."[28]

Warren and Halstead were conscious that it was a delicate task for the RF to become involved in another country's health care system without their presence becoming invasive, raising false hopes, or creating political turbulence. Their vision was a network whereby someone from the developing world would link up with someone from the developed world. Put them together, and they would find common objectives, with the ultimate aim of making the individual from the developing world, and the institution they represented, stronger. In a sense, programmes like INCLEN and the GND were a return to the foundation's missionary roots, only instead of bringing proven solutions to the unenlightened, Warren and

---

[26]Scott Halstead, personal communication.
[27]Gerald Keusch, personal communication.
[28]Scott Halstead, personal communication.

Halstead wanted to provide access to the intellectual tools that would enable people in developing countries to define and solve their own problems. Scott Halstead's realistic objectives for the clinical epidemiology network were clearly expressed in a letter to Walter Spitzer, professor of epidemiology and health at McGill University: "We hope INCLEN will help physicians in the poorest countries to see that their efforts need to be directed at alleviating and preventing priority health care problems. Under conditions of severe constraint, such as Ethiopia, the ability to respond to this message is limited. A second objective of INCLEN is to help hospital-based academic physicians to be better colleagues of preventive medicine and public health groups. We have to stifle our own urges and those of others, to see INCLEN as a total salvation. It is not. A lot of other pieces are needed to make the whole."[29]

Halstead's objectives at INCLEN, building on the work already done by White, had a clear and beneficial impact when put into practice in the field. In Thailand, a partnership between the RF and various health projects had existed for more than a century from a programme to combat hookworm to the establishment of a GND unit at Mahidol University in the 1970s under the leadership of Yongyuth Yuthavong. The country became an important and successful member of INCLEN, and the medical scientist, Prawase Wasi, wrote in glowing terms of Warren and Halstead's work: "I had the privilege of working with these two great men on this project. The initiative aimed to train clinicians in medical schools to focus more on epidemiology factors affecting clinical issues. The objective was to introduce population-based medicine into the thinking and practice of the medical schools to prepare them for future health system reform. In addition to the many health systems and medical training initiatives, the Foundation also supported the establishment of the National Epidemiological Board (NEB) in the Ministry of Public Health. A project initiated by Scott B. Halstead, who served as Associate Director of Health Science, the NEB became a national forum leading to health systems reform conceptualisation and development."[30] Few within the global health community would dispute that Warren played an important role in reactivating interest in neglected tropical diseases and in epidemiology in developing countries through his support for the INCLEN network.[31]

As with the GND, part of INCLEN's success was due to the atmosphere and operational ethos of the RF in the 1970s into the early 1980s. Warren, White, and Halstead's practical approaches to philanthropy in the field of tropical medicine reinforced the activist mentality of Frederick T. Gates, who sought practical solutions to public problems. When John Knowles, then the foundation president, had recruited Warren in 1977, this activist mentality still prevailed. New appointments formed a continuation of the foundation's original policy of placing professionals as

---

[29]Letter from S. Halstead to W. Spitzer, RF Archive, RF.88007 al 61, 21 February 1981.

[30]P. Wasi, Foreword in W. H. Becker, *Innovative Partners: The Rockefeller Foundation and Thailand (The RF centennial series)*, 2013, pp. 26–7.

[31]Brian Greenwood, personal communication.

administrators of philanthropic programmes. It was therefore not unusual for an M. D. to be hired to head the foundation's work in a specific area. During the 1970s and 1980s, for instance, Howard Klein was Director of Arts and Humanities at the RF. As a pianist, with two degrees from the Juilliard School of Music, and a former music critic for the New York Times, he too reinforced the foundation's belief in selecting professionals as administrators. He was part of the RF's inner-circle and an objective eyewitness to how strategies evolved and how they played out: "Knowles, even during his somewhat embattled period with the board of trustees who were perhaps made uncomfortable by his bravura style, continued to stress programmatic development based on keen analysis of problems and clearly defined solutions. He obviously brought Ken to the Foundation to do precisely what he did… I think it underlies Ken's freedom to act, a freedom that was key to his successes."[32] With the death of John D. Rockefeller III in 1978, however, the dynamics of the foundation's ethos began to change, a process that was accelerated by Knowles's death a year later. He was succeeded by Richard Lyman, an esteemed administrator, and a former president of Stanford, but unfortunately for Warren, not an internationalist.[33] The appointment of Lyman marked a transition away from using field professionals as administrators to hiring administrators with academic backgrounds to operate programmes. Had this seismic shift happened a decade earlier, Warren—and perhaps Knowles—might not have been recruited, or if hired, according to his colleague Howard Klein, "he might not have been allowed to cut the amazing swath in the field that his programmes did."[34]

Lyman's appointment heralded an era of sweeping change at the RF. In 1985, he hired the acclaimed American academic, Kenneth Prewitt, as a vice president, with the remit to design a new strategy for the science programmes. This allowed Lyman to concentrate on the aspects of the foundation's work in which he was profoundly interested: the civil rights programme, social justice, and the humanities. The division of labour worked well because Lyman didn't get along particularly well with Warren, but Prewitt did, and during the next few years Prewitt "protected" the Population, Health and Agricultural status quo and secured INCLEN's budget.[35] However, the forces of discontent were growing; the trustees and others were becoming restive with programmes that had been running for almost a decade. They wanted new projects to talk about that would provide a sense of renewal and a way to make their own indelible mark rather than merely rubberstamping on-going programmes. Lyman was uncomfortable with dynamic programme officers, the so-called "grand dukes" of the Federation,[36] and Scott Halstead was in no doubt that having a president who was not an internationalist and not a scientist led

[32]Howard Klein, personal communication.

[33]Kenneth Prewitt, personal communication.

[34]Howard Klein, personal communication.

[35]Kenneth Prewitt, personal communication.

[36]Howard Klein, personal communication.

directly to the RF distancing itself from continuing to financially support INCLEN.[37]

INCLEN, or a manifestation of it, still exists, with an office in India, but it is not the enlightened humanitarian organisation that Kerr White launched in 1980. Inimitable to both the GND and INCLEN were the meetings, and as soon as the RF quit, the meetings disappeared, and without them it was difficult to maintain the distinctive camaraderie and fellowship that characterised the project.[38] Both programmes thrived on the sense of excitement and fun at the meetings, of holding out goals for institutions and individuals, offering opportunities for both research and training that wouldn't have been otherwise available. The precarious nature of the funding was all the more disappointing because the RF had formed an historical link with both Warren and Halstead. Their respective careers in schistosomiasis and dengue had been supported by the foundation while they had met, befriended, and collaborated with other RF-sponsored scientists. Collectively they formed part of its scientific mission as established by John D. Rockefeller.[39] Yet times changed, and the relationship between the RF, Warren, and his colleagues and staff was being reconfigured. The clinical epidemiology programme had lasted a little more than a decade instead of becoming the generational-length programme that Halstead had envisaged.[40]

INCLEN graduates have populated, and often led, programmes that amalgamated clinical medicine and public health and fostered a well-informed understanding of the evidence base for medical decisions, which has come to be called "evidence-based medicine." This cohort of noteworthy individuals include, amongst others, Srinath Reddy, formally a cardiologist at the All India Institute of Medical Sciences and current President of the Public Health Foundation of India and Shally Awasthi, who was the lead researcher on DEVTA, the world's largest randomised controlled drug trial. This trial was published in 2013 and was dedicated to Ken Warren. Awasthi has also served on an international committee convened by the *Lancet* to propose reforms to medical education. Graduates of INCLEN have also served at the WHO in Geneva and have been Ministers of Health in Africa. Charles Karamagi, an INCLEN graduate from Uganda, established a graduate degree programme for physicians throughout Sub-Saharan Africa. The dean of the Medical School in Uganda, Nelson Sewankambo, was INCLEN-trained at McMaster. Arturo Morillo, a neurologist and dean of Columbia's leading medical school, was an early adopter of clinical epidemiology and became the director of INCLEN, encouraging its growth throughout Latin America.

---

[37]Scott Halstead, personal communication.

[38]$150,000 had been set aside for the annual INCLEN meeting to be held in Goa, India, January 22–29, 1989.

[39]*The Rockefeller Foundation 1913–1988*, The Rockefeller Foundation, p. 4.

[40]Scott Halstead, personal communication.

Short-lived it may have been, but short-sighted it wasn't. Chris Murray witnessed some of INCLEN's extraordinary contributions to human development: "I went to three or four meetings of INCLEN in the late 80s and early 90s and saw an incredible community building of people doing clinical epidemiology. I think when Rockefeller pulled out of funding it, INCLEN effectively collapsed, and nothing has come to fill that space. For a long period after the collapse of INCLEN, it was not at all fashionable to invest in training people, and so you saw a big scale-up of money for the AIDS emergency, PEPFAR, with almost nothing going into capacity building and training, and now the pendulum has moved back. People now recognise that you can't have an emergency for twenty years; you actually must take a longer term view, and you need to train scientists. Now capacity building is back [in a small way] but there has been nothing like INCLEN. If it [INCLEN] had kept going, I suspect it could have been better and better. I think what happened was that such a huge fraction of the budget at Rockefeller was going into sustaining INCLEN, that whoever was in charge at Rockefeller for Health [found that] there wasn't much room left to do anything, and it was very hard in the short-run to see the payoff from year to year."[41]

Unfortunately, the RF cut off funding for INCLEN before it had reached its full potential, and it has proved difficult to mobilise funding for the network's infrastructure from other sources. INCLEN still exists, based in India, but it is without the resources to maintain a truly international organisation. Furthermore, something of its lost potential can be measured by the programmes it germinated. China has established a national programme in clinical epidemiology originally inspired and led by INCLEN graduates. In the Philippines and elsewhere, INCLEN graduates have established the next generation of clinical epidemiology training centres in other medical schools in the region. INCLEN graduates have been active in the Cochrane Collaboration, helping the Cochrane address health problems of the developing world that might otherwise have been overlooked. In addition, INCLEN research groups, representing many countries in the less-developed world, have studied infectious diseases in children and family violence and have published their work in major international journals. As Kerr White, the creator of INCLEN wrote, "they have advanced understanding of the benefits of medical interventions in relation to their hazards and costs."

A major objective of INCLEN was to stimulate critical thinking about the behavioural aspect of disease prevention. Whether it was non-communicable or contagious diseases in developing countries, there were all sorts of problems to be solved, and every one of them was to some degree an economic, scientific, or educational challenge. What Halstead sought to do was to strengthen and advance the ideas of what became known as evidence-based medicine, i.e., to show how to collect and digest evidence, to ask what are the rules of evidence, and to show how to use statistics: This was the essence of the clinical epidemiology programme. Halstead remains resolute in his belief that the opportunity to build a lasting

---

[41]Christopher Murray, personal communication.

infrastructure for research and capacity building between rich and poor countries
was lost as INLCEN was prematurely wound up: "INCLEN died too early, and the
world is still floundering. If we had been in the thirtieth year of INCLEN there
would be a much stronger global research base. The world would have been a better
place if INCLEN had survived."[42]

Tropical Medicine

Warren's main preoccupation in life was tropical disease, yet while he could write
in 1981 that "above all, I consider myself a tropical medicine man," he believed the
term "tropical medicine" was in urgent need of redefinition. By the 1970s, few
people were writing about tropical medicine, and Warren believed that the term had
taken on negative connotations: If it was going to move with the times, he needed to
elevate its standing in the US. For Warren, "geographic medicine" was a more
accurate and less tendentious description of the subject and, crucially, that it should
be situated in departments of medicine so it was not divorced from clinical skills.[43]

In 1974, Warren became the first director of a Division of Geographic Medicine
in the US, a position made possible with a $525,000 grant from the RF.[44] Four
years later, the evolving concept was given further impetus when he co-authored,
with Adel Mahmoud, *Geographic Medicine for the Practitioner*, offering optimal
diagnostic methods and treatment of the so-called exotic diseases that affected
millions of travellers and migrants each year. Both men recognised that although
the scientific capacity of the developing world was increasing, scientists and
physicians in the developed world still had a role to play. This led them to co-edit
their encyclopaedic 1175-page *Tropical and Geographical Medicine* in 1984,
which remains a testament to their ideals and the concept of what today is
increasingly known as global health. In the preface to the textbook—which they
saw as providing a balanced guide for the student, the scientist, and the clinician—
the men also addressed the evolving nature of the subject: "In the last several
decades the practice of tropical and geographical medicine has undergone a drastic
change. The field essentially arose in Europe. Since World War II, however, there

---

[42]Scott Halstead, personal communication.

[43]The debate started at Case Western Reserve University Medical School when Dr Charles
Carpenter was appointed Chairman of Medicine and Physician-in-Chief. He asked Warren to
develop a division within the Department of Medicine to deal with infectious diseases in the
developing world. Dr Carpenter, a cholera expert, thought that the term "tropical medicine" in the
US did not have a good reputation, that it consisted of a few individuals who had little experience
of working in the tropics, and that "geographic medicine" would have wider appeal. Because the
term "geographic medicine" had been used some years earlier at NIH, the decision was to name the
new division "Geographic Medicine." According to Adel Mahmoud, "that is how the modern use
of the term started and we use it to say it is a new wave".

[44]MEDLINES to Case Western Reserve School of Medicine. January 1974, p. 1.

has been a remarkable burgeoning of medical schools throughout the tropical areas of Latin America, Africa, the Middle East and Asia. These schools, which have recognised the necessity of training their students to deal with their indigenous diseases, have increased the need for a general reference book."[45]

It was undoubtedly the case that the British experience of tropical medicine was very different in its evolution from that experienced by the US. In the US, there hadn't been the same colonial and missionary elements at play. For the Americans, tropical medicine was often a byproduct of fighting wars, and there was no tradition of sending medics to the tropics for decades at a time. Although both Mahmoud and Warren had attended the London School of Hygiene and Tropical Medicine, their earlier educational backgrounds were very different, with Mahmoud's foreshadowed by the death of his father when he was 10 years old, and the anti-imperialist Egyptian Revolution of 1952 led by Gamal Abdel Nasser. Mahmoud, who was born in 1941, attended the Cairo Medical School, an institution in a period of transition being run by the first generation of Egyptians after the "Brits" had left.[46] Cairo University Medical School was seen at the time as being one of the best in Africa, but when Mahmoud was a student there (1957–1963), the colonial penumbra was still in evidence. He remembers that Egyptians' main task was to "prove that they were better than their predecessors. Most of them had studied in England and their spoken English was very correct. It was known that if you used an Arabic word in your oral examination, you failed. This was difficult, because in the clinical examination you talked to the patient in Arabic, and you presented the case in English."[47] This background of attempting to distance the discipline from the colonial era heavily influenced Warren and Mahmoud's writing, and the textbook was very well received within the international health community. David Warrell, an infectious disease physician and an editor of the Oxford Textbook of Medicine, described it as "a classic" and that Mahmoud was "a kindred spirit" of Ken Warren "in creating a new excitement about Tropical Medicine."[48] Another leading British physician and communicable disease epidemiologist, David Bradley, thought that Warren and Mahmoud had written "the first modern American textbook of tropical medicine; a good one that freed itself from the traditional colonial image."[49] The book placed a new emphasis on mechanisms and pathogenesis of disease rather than on clinical presentation and therapy. As Warren and Mahmoud explained in their introduction, "the basic structure of the book reflects an understanding of all infectious agents as parasites in the broad sense of

---

[45]K. S. Warren & A. A. F. Mahmoud, *Tropical and Geographical Medicine*, McGraw-Hill, 1984, p. xvii.

[46]Adel Mahmoud, personal communication.

[47]Adel Mahmoud, personal communication.

[48]David Warrell, personal communication.

[49]David Bradley, personal communication.

the term. It presents the three crucial facets of the relationship between the infectious agent and the host: the parasite, the patient and the population."[50]

Transfer of Knowledge

Inseparable from the ideals of tropical and geographic medicine was Warren's determination to provide core libraries and information systems for medical schools and ministries of health in the developing world. He was equally resolute that he did not want to export to those destinations the indigestible behemoth of the medical and scientific information systems that had evolved as a stultifying accompaniment to Western-style medicine. This exacting realisation became self-evident through his own research on the history of schistosomiasis. The study began in 1967 with the publication of a complete computerised biography of schistosomiasis that included 10,286 references from 119 countries in 24 different languages covering a period of 110 years.[51] The compendium did not turn out to be as useful as Warren had expected: Only 30% of the studies were read one or more times and 15% twice or more. As a result, a core literature of approximately 400 studies was then established from those read six or more times. As a means of filtering out studies that were either wantonly esoteric, ephemeral, or of poor methodological design, Warren, working with his colleague William Goffman, an expert in information theory, applied a four-stage mathematical model considering the information system as a cyclic biologic process. This placement of selective filters at strategic points in the cycle, according to Warren, "was found to enhance the efficiency and quality of the system."[52] The exponential growth of the scientific literature made Warren believe that selectivity was obligatory. He was convinced, and had the biometric evidence to prove it, that although most physicians had insatiable and indiscriminate appetites for all biomedical information, most writers were deficient, and only 10% might be considered to be competent, with a far smaller number being major contributors.[53] He held particular distain for the paper that was never cited but was archived in perpetuity. This was another arena in which Warren was to have great influence, namely, measuring the impact of biomedical literature. Together with William Goffman, he performed a biometric study of the RF's GND programme, and although the different publications from the different units were

---

[50]K. S. Warren & A. A. F. Mahmoud, *Tropical and Geographical Medicine*, McGraw-Hill, 1984, p. xvii.

[51]K. S. Warren & V. A. Newill, *Schistosomiasis*: *A Bibliography of the World's Literature From 1852 to 1962*. 2 vols. Cleveland: The Press of Western Reserve University, 1967.

[52]K. S. Warren, "The Evolution of Selective Biomedical Libraries and Their Use in the Developing World." *JAMA*, 15 May 1987; Vol. 257, No 19, 2628–2629.

[53]K. S. Warren, "Selective aspects of the biomedical literature," in K. S. Warren (ed.), *Coping With the Biomedical Literature*: *A Primer for Scientists and Clinicians*. New York, Praeger Publishers, 1981, pp. 3–16.

very variable, it was nevertheless an attempt to evaluate impact.[54] Goffman defined biometrics as "the statistical analysis of published literature," and that the "purpose of the study is to aid in assessing the impact of this programme on the advancement of knowledge in these fields."[55]

Warren recognised, however, that although the affluent West could maintain its vast libraries, libraries were in catastrophic state in the developing world. Among the complications holding back efforts to obtain the most advanced medical information anywhere in the world were the problems of poverty, logistics, and intransigence. This was certainly the experience of David Bradley, who while working in East Africa made several attempts to ship medical books and journals from England but was thwarted by either recalcitrant universities reluctant to share the resource with other institutions or by bureaucratic torpor.[56] The disastrous situation was graphically depicted at a conference held by the RF in Bellagio, Italy, in 1979 on the theme of Selective Libraries for Medical Schools in Less-Developed Countries. Very little to ameliorate the situation was performed until 1985, when Scott Halstead, on discovering that the quality of microfiche readers had greatly increased, initiated a project to provide sites in the developing world with selected medical libraries on microfiche. With the assistance of University Microfilms Inc., many journals were made available on a quarterly basis, and a library was installed at Gadhaj Mada University, Indonesia.[57] Warren was hugely encouraging of his colleague's scheme because it resonated with his own continuing aim for the developing world to have access to medical information of high quality at low cost.

An opportunity to further cultivate this aim appeared at a chance meeting with Iain Chalmers at Bellagio in 1987. Chalmers, along with Murray Enkin and Mark Kires, his co-editors on what would become *A Guide to Effective Care in Pregnancy and Childbirth*, a two-volume systematic review of the randomised trials of obstetric care, were at Bellagio as part of a writers' residency. One evening they presented their work to the other guests, and afterward Warren came over to talk to them. Chalmers takes up the story: "Ken was very excited by our work and asked if he could help. Murray told him that we wanted to get this information out to women using the maternity services, but that they wouldn't even be able to lift the book, let alone use it in a practical way. Ken's reply was 'right, I'll give you $10,000 towards that.' This made it possible to produce a condensed version of the work, and that paperback is now in its fourth edition. We later started to publish electronically as well, as the Oxford database of perinatal trials started publishing in 1988, and that was something that intrigued Ken [too]."[58] At the same time, back at his Oxford base, Chalmers and his public health physician colleague, Muir Grey,

---

[54]Keith McAdam, personal communication.

[55]K. S. Warren & C. C. Jimenez (eds), *The Great Neglected Diseases of Mankind Biomedical Research Network: 1978–1988*. New York: The Rockefeller Foundation, 1988, p. 3.

[56]David Bradley, personal communication.

[57]Scott Haldane, personal communication.

[58]Sir Iain Chalmers, personal communication.

had discussed the problem of how to get the most accurate and effective medical information to even the most isolated parts of the world. Both men had a shared interest in the College of Medicine in Juba in Southern Sudan, yet each recognised that to get a copy of *The Lancet* to Juba would really be a substantial exercise involving a 10-day boat journey from Khartoum. Instead of seeking a conventional solution, their thoughts turned to the heavens. They envisioned a system whereby a communications satellite would be launched into orbit, and on the ground a Land Rover would pull up in some isolated part of the developing world, a laptop would be attached to the vehicle's battery, and as the satellite passed over, the latest copy of a medical journal could be pulled down. In this way the most advanced and up-to-date information would be accessible to all regardless of weather conditions or geographical location.[59]

These events were taking place in an increasingly febrile geopolitical world. Warren's generation had lived through the Cuban Missile Crisis of 1962, the hottest episode in the Cold War, when the United States and the Soviet Union came closest to nuclear warfare. It was a generation brought up on books such as *On Nuclear Warfare* and *Thinking the Unthinkable* and who had lived with the possibility of imminent nuclear war and the real fear as to whether survival was possible or even worthwhile.[60] Attempts had been made by the medical profession to restore a sense of shared humanitarianism to the Cold War stalemate, and as one of the world's leading advocates for the potential of vaccines to transform health, Warren was of great interest to a group of politicians and scientists who believed that if a channel of communication and trust could be established between biomedical scientists in the United States and in the Soviet Union, then a great collaborative enterprise might be created to improve the health of people throughout the world. John Dingell, the former Democratic member of the House of Representatives and the Chairman of the Committee on Energy and Commerce, employed a number of people, including the renowned researchers Phyllis Freeman and Anthony Robbins, to develop possible areas of collaboration. They had the idea that harnessing the collective might of the Soviet Union and the US could provide all of the much needed vaccines for all of the diseases in the developing world, and as such, Warren was one of their first ports of call.[61]

The ever-increasing interconnectivity of the political and scientific worlds was bolstered by the founding, in 1980, of the International Physicians for the Prevention of Nuclear War (IPPNW), an action that formed a step-change in the

---

[59]Sir Iain Chalmers, personal communication.

[60]G. Weissmann, *The Woods Hole Cantata: Essays on the Science and Society.* Houghton Mifflin Company Boston, 1985.

[61]Anthony Robbins, personal communication. A. Robbins & P. Freeman, "Obstacles to Developing Vaccines for the Third World," *Scientific American,* Vol. 256, No. 11, pp. 126–233, 1988; *Proceedings of a Workshop on Vaccine Innovation and Supply.* Report prepared by the Institute of Medicine National Academy of Sciences for the use of the Subcommittee on Oversight and Investigations of the Committee on Energy and Commerce. US Government Printing Office. 1986.

profession's influence.[62] The organisation was established to bridge the east–west political divide and to educate the public about the medical consequences of nuclear war. The IPPNW was a non-partisan organisation with two of its leading figures being the legendary cardiologists Bernard Lown and Yevgeniy Chazov. It had an immediate and catalysing effect on the medical profession world-wide as well as on American politics, and Warren was immediately drawn into its orbit. Over the next couple of years, Warren and Robbins began to work directly with the IPPNW, seeing its power and influence grow as its membership reached 135,000 across 41 countries. In parallel, the resurgence of the American Republican Party under the leadership of Ronald Reagan, who became President in January 1981, resulted in the launch of an idea for the Strategic Defense Initiative. This futuristic vision of a satellite early-warning system allied to ballistic missiles—Reagan's Buck Rogers fantasies for outer space—once again heightened the fear of nuclear warfare and became universally known as "Star Wars."[63] This concept was anathema to Bernard Lown, who envisioned satellite technology being deployed to enhance human health rather than to destroy it. Lown suggested the creation of a satellite-based global health-communications system as a means of showing that space could unite rather than divide the world. This portentous idea, which bore clear similarities to Chalmers and Grey's musings on the topic, was recognised by Anthony Robbins, who would later become IPPNW's treasurer, as an important vision: "Bernie Lown came up with a brilliant idea, which was really a part of a political strategy of how to deal with the nuclear arms race and all of the technology around it. He came up with 'SatelLife,' which was a scheme that used the satellites that had become central to nuclear weapons, and which were capable of anything and everything, and to use these same low-orbit satellites for peaceful purposes."[64] The peaceful objectives were to improve communications and exchanges of information in the fields of public health with a special emphasis on areas of the world which were restricted by poor communications, wars, or natural disasters. Moreover, such ideas were given extra kudos when, in 1985, the IPPNW was awarded the Nobel Peace Prize. The Nobel Committee noted IPPNW's role in "opposition to the proliferation of atomic weapons and to a redefining of priorities, with greater attention being paid to health and other humanitarian issues."[65]

---

[62]In 1951, in Britain, Lionel Penrose, Horace Joules, Ian Gilliland, Richard, and Joan Doll co-founded the Medical Association for the Prevention of War (MAPW). This scientific alliance pre-dated the Russell–Einstein Manifesto, which was established in 1955 when the Cold War was at its most intense. The MAPW announced its existence on 20th January 1951 in a letter to *The Lancet*: "We appeal to our fellow doctors who think there may yet be an alternative to merely providing treatment for casualties; we ask them to join us, in the spirit of our chosen profession of healing, in doing all in their power to halt preparation for war and to bring about a new and determined approach to the peaceful settlement of disputes and to world disarmament."

[63]G. Weissmann, *The Woods Hole Cantata, Essays on Science and Society*, New York, 1985, p. 121.

[64]Anthony Robbins, personal communication.

[65]In Oslo on 10 December 1985, Bernard Lown and Yevgeniy Chazov accepted the Nobel Prize on behalf of their colleagues.

Ken Warren was immediately intrigued with the SatelLife idea because he knew that poverty of information was a significant obstacle to better health in the developing world. Moreover, he had established close links with the National Library of Medicine and the British Library, which would theoretically enable SatelLife to create a reservoir of information for use across the globe. Throughout the 1980s, Warren advised the IPPNW on the development of the scheme and attended the IPPNW's Seventh World Congress in Moscow in 1987, which attracted more than 2000 physicians from 70 countries. Robbins recognised that SatelLife now required an expert custodian to guide its progress; accordingly he hired Charlie Clements to direct the project and put Ken Warren on its board.

Bernard Lown, although a brilliant cardiologist and a man of incredible focus, had no knowledge of the developing world. Indeed, whereas the Nobel Prize had highlighted the conversation between the East and West about the dangers of nuclear war, the global South was totally ignored in that conversation. Warren intended to ensure that the South would not be neglected, and had a profound understanding of the impact that the medical information delivered by SatelLife technology could have on health care systems. He launched himself wholeheartedly into the project, taking direct action, and in addition to occupying a place on the Board of SatelLife, he also helped to raise money for the cosmic experiment.

The satellites, containing a computer and radio, were built by Surrey Satellite Technology Ltd, in the UK, at the University of Surrey in England. The first of the two, HealthSat 1, was launched in 1991, and HealthSat II was launched in 1993. Each satellite, approximately the same shape and size of a domestic refrigerator, circumnavigated the poles and was capable of reaching every part of the earth four times daily. The idea was that the satellite would circle the earth many times a day, changing its flight-path slightly, and as it went over a computer connected to a radio, it would send down the message "Do you have outgoing mail today?" Essentially, it could get emails to places in remotest Africa that did not have telephone connections in an era before the Internet. Originally, the Soviet Union had promised SatelLife free launches, but given the internal collapse of the Communist Party, the launches were undertaken by the French Aerospace Agency in the South Pacific.

The project was pioneered in five East African countries: Kenya, Uganda, Tanzania, Zimbabwe, and Zambia. Within 5 years, SatelLife established email networks in the health sectors of 18 African countries approximately a decade before the Internet arrived, a remarkable achievement. Moreover, as Charlie Clements noted, "we had permission from over 60 journals to deliver their content to people in the developing world."[66] SatelLife was not only about delivering the most up-to-date information. It created an epidemiological early warning system so that parts of the network could alert their colleagues around the world when they were seeing things that they did not recognise, and in doing so, clearly echoed Warren, White, and Halstead's INCLEN project. By establishing digital

---

[66]Charlie Clements, personal communication.

communication in Africa at a very early, important stage, SatelLife represented an experimental advance and the expression of a humanitarian cause from which many in the developing world benefited. Charlie Clements worked closely with Warren in creating the global communications system and identifies the important role his colleague played in shaping its evolution: "Ken was a great promoter of SatelLife and helped us to raise money. He was a very enthusiastic man, and it could be contagious. He was a real visionary, and I think his GND campaign made Dr. Lown and Dr. Chazov aware that there was a neglected part of the world in the South. He led many in the world to think about those diseases."[67]

The IPPNW delegates attending the Seventh World Congress in Moscow in 1987 may have felt a sense of excitement at the prospect that they might help bring peace to the world. Ken Warren's focus was not entirely the same as the IPPNW's, although he certainly supported the cause. Conversely, some of the delegates may, with a resigned sense of detachment, have believed that in 1987 the human race was living on borrowed time.[68] Warren's own career trajectory bore poignant parallels: His professional achievements in the decade since being appointed the RF's Director of Health Sciences had been prodigious, but now oppositional forces were gathering, and he too was living on borrowed time.

---

[67]Charlie Clements, personal communication.

[68]In 1991, Kurt Vonnegut in his book, *Fates Worse than Death* wrote, "My guess is that... we really will blow up everything by and by."

Chapter 5
The Fall

In 1986, Warren received a letter from Professor W.W. "Bill" Macdonald, Dean of the Liverpool School of Tropical Medicine, informing him that he was to be awarded the Mary Kingsley Medal,[1] the school's highest award, "in recognition of your outstanding contributions to the improvement of health in the developing world."[2] Warren was to share the award with Adetokunbo O. Lucas of the Carnegie Corporation and former director of the TDR. A decade earlier, in 1976, Lucas, as Director of the WHO's programme on Tropical Diseases Research, produced a programme that comprised six groups of diseases: malaria, schistosomiasis, the filariases (including onchocerciasis and lymphatic filariasis), the trypanosomiases (African sleeping sickness and Chagas disease), the leishmaniasis, and leprosy. Warren had criticised the inclusion of some of these diseases and the omission of others, which he saw as posing a greater health burden. Scott Halstead, Warren's deputy at the RF, notes that Warren's circumspection was not a consequence of personal dynamics but rather was institutional in origin. "Ken was never very comfortable or happy with TDR. I think he saw it as competition and viewed it as a mini NIH with the strengths and weaknesses of NIH."[3]

On the bottom of the letter from Macdonald, Warren wrote his reply, which indicated that there had been a mellowing of any sense of competition that may have existed between the two men and their parallel programmes: "That Dr. A.O. Lucas will be receiving the medal also only increases my good feelings about the occasion. We have both been working toward the same goals within very different

---

[1]The medal commemorates the remarkable Mary Kingsley who left Liverpool in 1893 to explore West Africa. She was the author of the renowned book *Travels in West Africa*, which vividly described the realities of life in the tropics to succeeding generations.

[2]Letter from W .W. Macdonald to K. S. Warren, New York, 23 June 1986. Courtesy of Sylvia Warren.

[3]Scott Halstead, personal communication.

© Springer International Publishing AG 2017   105
C. Keating, *Kenneth Warren and the Great Neglected Diseases*
of Mankind Programme, Springer Biographies,
DOI 10.1007/978-3-319-50147-5_5

institutions. I certainly feel that our efforts would have been far less successful without his hard work and great accomplishments."[4]

Although plaudits were never in short supply in recognition of Warren's pivotal role shaping some of the most important campaigns to reduce the global burden of disease, the 1986 award foreshadowed the end of his tenure at the RF. During the past decade, Warren had become a dynamic programme officer, one of the foundation's "Grand Dukes" who thrived in the highly charged and competitive atmosphere as both a grant-giver and a mobiliser of funding.[5] He had survived the death of his mentor, John Knowles, and had ridden out the storm that arrived with the appointment of Richard Lyman as president, but the arrival of a new chair of the trustees in 1987 was to prove terminal for Warren's Rockefeller career. There were, of course, mitigating issues. International health, as envisaged by Knowles and Warren, was in the process of being downgraded by the foundation. There was also a growing antipathy to Warren's autonomous, if innovative, management style and, conceivably, his inability to adapt to, or even fully comprehend, the change of philanthropic direction that made his situation vulnerable. Tellingly, Warren's Grants Secretary, Orneata Prawl, who worked closely with him, identified a defect in his managerial style that weakened his position within the foundation: "Ken Warren was brilliant, but the one problem was, playing politics was not his strong suit. Ken was very direct about his expectations, but did not handle the politics well."[6] Although Warren had spent much of his scientific life surrounded by the politics of international health, he was not always a skilled operator when it came to dealing with the "people politics" of the RF's upper echelons.

With the internal dynamics of the RF changing, the programmes that Warren had championed, and even his own role, came under greater scrutiny. Previously, he occupied the status of the quintessential programme officer, which, according to Howard Klein, Head of Arts, "made Ken a forceful advocate for his programmes and positions. Ken was a star, the right person at the right time."[7] Warren was an entrepreneur, an impresario defending his grantees and holding the Health Sciences Division together in a style that the medical historian William Muraskin described as a "type of free-wheeling, autonomous visionary."[8] Yet although Warren's colleagues noted that he had a big heart and was charming and charismatic, his personality could divide opinion. As his Grants Secretary remembers, "you either accepted Ken the way he was, or you disliked him. I cannot actually say whether people liked Ken Warren, I think they respected him. And that is a big difference."[9]

---

[4]Letter from W. W. Macdonald to K. S. Warren, New York, 23 June 1986. Courtesy of Sylvia Warren.

[5]Howard Klein, personal communication.

[6]Orneata Prawl, personal communication.

[7]Howard Klein, personal communication.

[8]W. Muraskin, *The Politics of International Health. The Children's vaccine initiative and the struggle to develop vaccines for the Third World.* State University of New York Press. 1998, p. 159.

[9]Orneata Prawl, personal communication.

Certainly Warren could be brusque, immodest, and ostentatious, which coupled with a single-mindedness that blinded him to problems and obstacles along the way, coalesced to ferment a sense of ambivalence in those who could otherwise have become his defenders. As the malariologist Louis Miller noted, Warren's personality showed simultaneously strength of character combined with the weakness of not knowing when to be reticent: "if someone attacked him he did not know how to deflect them, but continued to come back for more fight."[10] This observation accurately reflects the dissonance between the prodigious accomplishments of Warren's professional life and the complex psychology which drove it. This did not necessarily bode well for Warren in a time of change (Fig. 5.1).

The arrival at the RF of Kenneth Prewitt in 1985 allowed Warren to continue to pursue his ideals under the Science Based Development programme. Driving Warren's policy forward was the idea of mobilizing the science of industrialised countries on behalf of the developing world. This equipoise disappeared in 1987 with the arrival of John Evans as chair of the trustees. Evans, a Canadian, was a renaissance man; after winning a Rhodes scholarship at the University of Oxford, he trained as a cardiologist, earning the reputation as an "extraordinary physician and leader."[11] Later he joined the World Bank where he was the founding director of the organisation's Population, Health and Nutrition Department. As a politician, business leader, and educator, so garlanded was his life that one obituary notice recorded that "it would be impossible to overstate the contribution of this remarkable man."[12] Evans was enormously respected by the other RF trustees thanks to his judicious demeanour, commanding presence, and knowledge of the medical world. One could be forgiven for thinking that because Evans and Warren were both medically orientated and had a mutual interest in improving health in the developing world, that all the constituent elements were in place to ensure a harmonious collaboration. However, Evans and Warren were not cut from the same cloth. In another obituary entry, the behavioural gulf dividing the men was put into stark contrast: "Keep your accomplishments to yourself." Evans advised his six children, "people don't like flash."[13] Although the two men were not necessarily kindred spirits, while Warren continued to deliver programmes that commanded the support of the president, political turbulence stayed at manageable levels. In 1988, however, Richard Lyman retired, and Peter Goldmark became the 11th president of the RF. Goldmark was interested in environmental issues, and his arrival ended the successful managerial division of labour that had existed at the foundation since 1985. During that period, Richard Lyman had devoted his attentions to the humanities and developing a special interest in civil rights, whereas Prewitt had

---

[10]Louis Miller, personal communication.

[11]Joe Cook, personal communication.

[12]Tamsin McMahon, *The Toronto Globe and Mail*, 13 February 2015.

[13]Judy Stoffman, *The Toronto Globe and Mail,* 6 March, 2015.

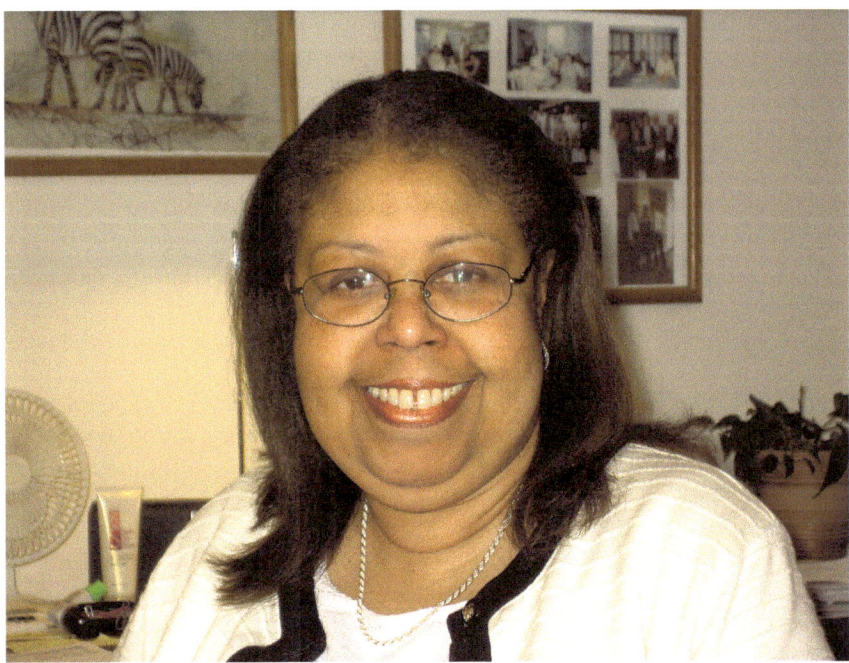

Fig. 5.1 Orneata Prawl, Ken Warren's Grants Secretary at the RF, and organiser of the final GND meeting, held in Kenya in 1987. Courtesy of Orneata Prawl

managed the scientific programmes, attending meetings, briefed the trustees, and ensured that Ken Warren, as well as his projects, were protected.[14]

Each presidential transition was marked by the ending of old programmes and the implementation of new projects as incoming incumbents aspired to leave their personal imprint on the foundation. John Evans and Peter Goldmark immediately formed an alliance based on a shared view of the future direction of the foundation. Together, the men believed that the foundation wasn't leaving the right kind of footprint in the developing world, that Health Sciences had been treated too much like royalty, and that Warren had been too elitist in his work as director.[15] Instead, they sought greater mobilisation and, by incorporating NGOs, to get back to the grass roots. Moreover, Goldmark believed that he had inherited a foundation that was a collection of independent fiefdoms and accordingly set in motion a process to centralise power and curb autonomy.[16] Ken Prewitt, who had seen himself as a friend and protector of Warren, now felt compromised for two reasons. First, he had

---

[14]Kenneth Prewitt, personal communication.

[15]Kenneth Prewitt, personal communication.

[16]W. Muraskin, *The Politics of International Health. The Children's vaccine initiative and the struggle to develop vaccines for the Third World.* State University of New York Press. 1998, p. 159.

been the internal candidate for the presidency, but the position went to Goldmark with the trustees' proviso that Prewitt would be kept on the payroll. The obvious combustible nature of such a power struggle at the apex of the foundation meant, according to Prewitt, that "we fought constantly."[17] Second, some of Warren's perceived financial extravagances—too many trips to Bellagio, exorbitant expense account, flights on the Concorde—were coming under greater scrutiny and were increasingly more difficult for Prewitt to defend to the new administration. Warren was unrepentant; he certainly didn't mind ruffling the feathers of the financial administrators if they queried a bill for a lavish dinner with scientific colleagues because he really did believe, as the directors in the 1920s did, that it was his foundation.

Another factor weakening Warren's power base was the intellectual sclerosis consuming the trustees, who were increasingly unexcited by the achievements of the GND programme and INCLEN, which had been the mainstays of the Health Sciences Division for almost a decade. Instead the trustees wanted new projects, new ideas to discuss, and a fresh sense of their own value. In John Evans they had a new leader who moved in medical circles and who had ideas, who wanted to roll up his sleeves, and who was determined to challenge the status quo. Alongside Goldmark, he was all too aware that the only way to ensure long-term interest in a policy was to readapt it to the changing times. Prewitt had proved to be a master at this, whereas Warren was uninterested in such semantics, prioritising instead good science and good people as the drivers of transformation. He certainly played politics well in the echelons of science, but he had bordering on contempt for people who didn't understand his vision for the Health Sciences Division. On the other hand, Evans—with a deep knowledge of health sciences and a reputation as one of the most celebrated medical educationalists of his generation—reacted against Warren's overt, and sometimes arrogant, confidence in science. Whereas Warren believed in elite institutions and elite scientists, Evans held that although the scientists in question may well have been world-leaders, rather than needing to know the detailed genomics of an obscure organism, more attention should be paid to the delivery of existing interventions. In essence it was almost a battle between primary health care and sophisticated science.

A further concern for Warren was that the GND, his flagship programme, was perceived to concentrate too much in the rich North to the detriment of the poor South. This, to some extent, was an inevitable criticism as the programme set out to bring the fruits of the new biology, genetics, and molecular biology to bear on tropical diseases. The laboratories to do this didn't exist to any great extent in the tropics, and as a consequence the scientific establishments of Harvard, the Karolinska Institute, and the University of Oxford were recruited in the initial first stage of the project. Nevertheless. of the 14 foundation units, only 3 were located in the South (Mexico, Thailand, and Egypt). This was seen as an important organisational shortcoming and one that left the programme open to criticism that it had

---

[17]Kenneth Prewitt, personal communication.

not established a truly reciprocal partnership between North and South. Unless there was emphasis on the receiving end as well as the sending end, so the argument ran, then only marginal health gains in the South would be made. As a colleague, Joyce Moock, who spent 28 years as a foundation officer, suggested, "if at the time, he [Warren] had invested more in the South … I think the programme may have gone on a bit longer."[18]

Warren had written that support for the GND programme would be for "at least eight years" and he succeeded in guiding it to that stated minimum, but not beyond.[19] The foundation had offered Warren a rare opportunity, but his leadership was dependent on his ability to successfully read the mood of the organisation and move with the changing times. Once he sensed the change in the mood music, Warren began to put together some ideas that might placate the Goldmark–Evans position. Accordingly, he contacted his friend, the immunologist Tore Godal, who became Director of the WHO's Tropical Diseases Research Programme (TDR) in 1986, with the idea of establishing a collaborative research programme to construct a global laboratory to study tropical diseases.[20] This joint venture uniting the two leading agencies in the field was looked upon in some quarters as ground-breaking. John David notes that "Ken started something once which was never done again and it was fabulous: he started to collaborate with TDR. There were mutual double grants … in which the developed countries got money from him and the developing countries got funding from the TDR as a matching grant. It was wonderful: it was a way of getting expertise for the developing world and also using developing world people. It made for a very good collaboration, and was never done again."[21] Alas, for Warren even this far-sighted initiative failed to remove the hesitancies that the foundation's hierarchy had about his stewardship. Indeed, far from liberating him, Warren's new plan, according to Godal, further exacerbated his situation: "There was a synergy between the GND and TDR and when I became Director in 1986, Ken invited me to go to his meetings and he suggested that we should partner, which I thought was a great idea. Then we could have both institutions in the North and institutions in the South. Because most of the TDR units were in the South, I suggested that the TDR should support the southern partners and Ken support the northern partner. And he agreed. But I think that marked the start of his end at the RF, because the board thought that Ken was consciously developing associations to support his friends [within the GND] but that was not the case."[22]

---

[18]Joyce Moock, personal communication.

[19]K. S. Warren & C. C. Jimenez (eds), *The Great Neglected Diseases of Mankind Biomedical Research Network: 1978–1988*. New York: The Rockefeller Foundation, 1988, p. 1.

[20]"The TDR-Rockefeller Foundation joint funding venture, announced last year, was seen as an important way to strengthen collaboration between different groups of research workers—to be backed by substantial R&D support. Over 200 'letters of intent' were submitted, and, of these, 29 have been invited to prepare formal proposals—although possibly no more than 10 will be selected for major funding". Parasitology Today, Vol 4, No 5, 1988, p. 123.

[21]John David, personal communication.

[22]Tore Godal, personal communication.

Just how tenuous Warren's hold on the division had become was immediately apparent to his closest friend, Adel Mahmoud, when Evans visited his laboratory at Case Western Reserve University. Mahmoud recounts that "I knew Ken was having difficulties with him, but Evans said to me 'the problem with what Ken is trying to do, is that it is too little, too late.' When the chair of the board of trustees says this, you are history."[23] As well as policy differences, Evans and Warren had strikingly different personalities, which led to tensions inside the RF's headquarters on Fifth Avenue. Orneata Prawl didn't think that Evans liked Warren, and that the "writing was on the wall for Ken."[24] Moving in medical circles, the probity-minded Evans may have become embarrassed when he heard Warren's detractors, of which there were a number, asking him how he could put up with someone like Ken Warren who appeared to be presumptuously living off the hog.[25] Inside the foundation there was a feeling that Warren's 35 visits to Bellagio were excessive, even though he had used it as a vehicle for some of the most successful health campaigns in the second half of the twentieth century.

Selective primary health care, which has now become the guiding principle for the WHO's integrated large-scale preventive treatment for control or elimination of NTDs, began life as a Bellagio conference. Likewise, Good Health Care at Low Cost, the theme of a meeting held at Bellagio between April 29 and May 3, 1985, became the philosophical cornerstone of the modern programme of mass drug administration, i.e., of doing something simple at a very high cost-effective ratio. Additionally, The Global Campaign to Immunise the World's Children, which took place in March 1984, established health priorities in the developing world that still resonate today. Warren's farsighted accomplishment was to exploit Bellagio's convening appeal to bring together researchers both from academia and the pharmaceutical companies to form lasting collaborations. These alliances were forerunners of the current Public Private Partnerships (PPPs) that are emblematic of modern strategies on tropical disease research.

It is undisputable that Warren used his visits to Bellagio to great effect. It was at the villa that a huge number of his greatest ideas, projects. and collaborations in health exploration were made. In fact, in recognition of his efforts, particularly relating to the Child Survival and Development Revolution, in 1988, James Grant, the Executive Director of UNICEF at that time, celebrated Warren's success at putting biomedical knowledge to use in the Third World: "The accelerated health programmes to which Ken Warren has contributed so much have brought a new political visibility, and consequently increased financial support, to Primary Health Care (PHC) and other programmes for children. It is the success of these politically

---

[23]Adel Mahmoud, personal communication.

[24]Orneata Prawl, personal communication.

[25]Ken Prewitt, personal communication.

attractive programmes which has contributed so much to getting children placed, for the first time, on the political agenda of various summit meetings."[26]

Yet even Warren's greatest supporters couldn't deny that there was a propensity for self-sabotage in his behaviour. He had a sense of entitlement that was ingrained,[27] and Prewitt believed that some of his injudicious expense account claims had "weakened his moral stature," while the perceived excesses of Bellagio were damaging.[28] Also, although Warren had learned to use his power in beneficial ways, there were some aspects of the power dynamic that he never quite understood. He sometimes forgot that just because he became persuaded of an idea, it did not mean that he had discovered it,[29] and he could become too enthralled with powerful individuals. This was certainly the case in the mid-1980s, when Warren set out to launch a health project in the Philippines at a time when the dictator Imelda Marcos was in power. Everyone should be on their guard when dictators are on a "charm" offensive. John Bruer was with Ken Warren on the evening that the red carpet was rolled out for Marcos' representatives at the Century Association in New York: "These guys walked in and I said, 'Ken, you cannot do business with these people, the bad that will come will far outweigh any good you could do for tropical medicine research in the Philippines. These people have questionable morals and are not above using you and the foundation for their own ends.' And Ken finally did see that one, but there was always this attraction to the powerful, and Ken sometimes held this in check and sometimes he didn't."[30]

Warren was fast approaching a major intersection in his career: Not only was he a convenient foil for Evans' wish to create a sense of departure from what had gone before, but a new generation of health specialists with persuasive ideas was entering the field. One celebrated member of that group was the epidemiologist Seth Berkley who—like Warren—was an advocate of the efficacious power of vaccines. Furthermore, his outstanding work in disease control in Brazil and Uganda had brought him to the attention of Ken Prewitt, who was determined to bring him to the foundation in a leadership role. Berkley had first met Warren in Bahia, Brazil, while studying tropical medicine and had a lot of respect for Warren's science: "He was a brilliant thinker, a strategic guy and an incredibly prolific guy. So he was impressive, he could be very arrogant, but arrogant in the way of 'the power of science and scientists.' I had been working in Uganda with Bill Foege on the Task Force for Child Survival all on the Rockefeller nickel. Then someone had the bright idea to say to the president, Peter Goldmark, 'there's a guy in Uganda who knows what's going on, why don't you go visit him?' So I took him [Goldmark] around

---

[26]J. Grant, Speech to the New York Academy of Sciences L. S. Fohlich Award Conference, 18 October 1988. Published by UNICEF.

[27]Orneata Prawl, personal communication.

[28]Ken Prewitt, personal communication.

[29]David Bradley, personal communication.

[30]John Bruer, personal communication.

out into the field, myself driving, which was a real experience. That was how I got to know the Rockefeller team well."[31]

The GND was the first attempt by a big philanthropic organisation to take on the global health agenda. It drew up a list of major infectious diseases and sought to get the best biomedical scientists from all over the world, experienced in sequential adaptive reasoning, to bear on these diseases.[32] Warren represented a link—ultimately the final link—in a historic chain going back to the inception of the RF, to the era of the Circuit Riders and the omnipotent, scientifically orientated Directors of Health. Also, the neuralgic personal atmosphere that existed between Evans and Warren was symptomatic of a deeper strategic rift, i.e., what was the role of the RF? Was it to push the boundaries of knowledge or was it to move toward being a more delivery-based organisation in the field? The RF had been a very science-based organisation, and Seth Berkely was aware of the friction between the two strategic positions. "Ken's belief in science led him to cross swords with John Evans, who was a powerful individual in the health field, so maybe that was a case of two alpha bulls in the same room. It became a battle between primary health care versus sophisticated science."[33] Eventually the indirect signalling from Evans to Ken Prewitt became so great that something had to give. Prewitt during this whole process had become a deft semiotician, deciphering the indirect messages, which—although never directly articulated—were clear: Get rid of Ken Warren.

Prewitt was not the first academic who needed to practice interpretation management while working for John Evans. Dean Jamison had a similar experience while working for Evans at the World Bank: "I knew Evans quite well, he was my boss for a couple of years, and it was pretty clear sometimes that I was supposed to do what he wanted me to do... And I thought it was completely his prerogative to tell me 'Dean, do it this way,' and I might disagree, we'd have an argument, and then we'd do it his way, and that's fine, that's how the process works... But what would piss me off was he would want *me* to decide to do it his way, and I used to get upset about that. I would happily do it his way if he told me to. But I wasn't going to go through the charade of agreeing with him about it. He was the boss, he decides and that's fine, that is the way the process works. I can empathise with Prewitt there."[34] Prewitt occupied the unenviable position of arbitrator-in-chief between foundation officers' destinies and the impulses of their bosses, and although he felt great loyalty to his friend Warren, he felt that the future lay with Berkley. With a sense of guilt over not being able to further protect his old colleague, Prewitt delivered the message.[35]

Warren spent the last of his 11 years at the Rockefeller as Associate Vice President for Molecular Biology and Information Science. The title recognised his

---

[31]Seth Berkley, personal communication.

[32]John Bell, personal communication.

[33]Seth Berkley, personal communication.

[34]Dean Jamison, personal communication.

[35]Kenneth Prewitt, personal communication.

innate interest in the subjects while accurately signposting the intellectual desti-
nation of his subsequent career. A further reason for the redeployment may have
been a genuine wish of the foundation to offer one of its most high-profile officers
the time to arrange a seamless transition that would maintain his credibility and
status,[36] thus allowing him the opportunity to clear his desk and leave the foundation with his head held high.[37] Unfortunately for Warren, this opportunity was
not afforded him. The beleaguered Health Sciences Division urgently needed a
charismatic figure who could devise approaches to a set of problems based on
research, someone who would be as forceful an advocate for its reasoned programmes as Warren had been. Regrettably, a full-time director of Health Sciences
was not appointed until 1991, 4 years after Warren had vacated the position, by
which time much of the productive work of the division had suffered. Scott
Halstead, not even considered by his superiors as a candidate to fill the permanent
position, became acting director, working alongside Ken Prewitt in the increasingly
listless division.[38] What seemed singularly punitive about the final year of Warren's
employment was the bureaucratic tactlessness with which he was treated. It was
decided that Warren was not to be moved, that he would stay within the precincts of
his old protectorate, the Health Sciences Division. There he would be subjected to
hearing its gossip, see his former grantees wandering through the corridors, and feel
the daily heat of humiliation. Orneata Prawl believes that the final year must have
been hard to endure for her former boss: "They gave him a Vice President title, but
as far as I was concerned it was meaningless, it had no substance behind it. They
treated it as if he had been promoted but I felt that he had been demoted. I would
prefer the clean cut and not to prolong the agony. But to put him on the same
floor... they could have done what they had done with other people, and pay them
to be a consultant and write their memoir off in an office someplace. But to have
him there at the foundation, I thought that it was not only awkward, I thought it was
cruel. And that was sad."[39]

Jerry Keusch believes that the way the Rockefeller dealt with Ken Warren was
"appalling" and the end was "tragic."[40] Scott Halstead remains "bitter" about the
way Warren was forced out, and that the ending of Warren's GND programme in
1988 was "criminal" and "stupid" given the list of stellar individuals and institutions it nurtured and developed.[41] Although Warren was frozen out of the foundation by its executive, acts of kindness by his colleagues softened the blow.
Excommunication was not total. Late in 1988, at a large meeting of the

---

[36]Kenneth Prewitt, personal communication.

[37]Joyce Moock, personal communication.

[38]W. Muraskin, *The Politics of International Health. The Children's vaccine initiative and the struggle to develop vaccines for the Third World.* State University of New York Press. 1998, p. 159.

[39]Orenata Prawl, personal communication.

[40]Gerald Keusch, personal communication.

[41]Scott Halstead, personal communication.

philanthropic glitterati in the foundation's headquarters, Ken and Sylvia were seated at a small table far-distant from the other senior foundation officers. Then, Adolfo Martinez-Palomo, a GND investigator at the National Polytechnic Institute in Mexico, walked over and joined them. Pulling up a chair, he spent the whole evening with Ken and Sylvia, refusing to take up his seat at the top table. Warren was deeply moved by this act of kindness; it was a recognition that although he was being ostracised institutionally, the atmosphere of friendly respect, redolent of the GND network, still endured.[42]

Soon the pungent aroma of Warren's cigars, which for years had permeated the offices of the entire Health Sciences Division would dissolve, and no longer would the sounds of Johann Sebastian Bach's *The Goldberg Variations* emanate from his office late in the evening. The Rockefeller years were the highpoint of Warren's professional life. When he left Cleveland for New York, he effectively ended his own career as a practitioner of science, however, in recompense he shaped the scientific lives of a generation spread across the world. Warren's legacy is the continuation of scientific research into the complex problems of parasitic diseases; we are, in some respects, still living his vision today. Yet, implausible as it may seem, the Rockefeller Foundation today does not have a recognisable health programme. The date of the foundation's decoupling from its core ideal—identifying disease as the supreme ill in human life—can be traced to a combination of the fall of Warren, managerial atrophy, and a failure to move with the times.[43] Ken Prewitt delineates the historical line that culminated in the decisive break with tradition: "I wish that I had fought harder, because if Ken had stayed he would have been formidable. If I had left him in place he would have redesigned things, but we lost three years of productive work. So health lost and it [the RF] never really got it back."[44]

Of course, it is not necessarily a bad thing to move on. All of us from time to time need a sense of renewal and natural progression. At least one of Warren's friends believed that he would simply look for other kingdoms to conquer.[45] Although Warren had lost his job, he retained his incisive mind and decisive

---

[42]Sylvia Warren, personal communication.

[43]In conjunction with *The Lancet*, the Rockefeller Foundation launched a new initiative on planetary health. In the final report of the Rockefeller Foundation-*Lancet* Commission on Planetary Health, this was defined as: "the achievement of the highest attainable standard of health, wellbeing, and equity worldwide through judicious attention to the human systems—political, economic, and social—that shape the future of humanity *and* the Earth's natural systems that define the safe environmental limits within which humanity can flourish. Put simply, planetary health is the health of human civilisation and the state of natural systems on which it depends." S. Whitmee, A. Haines, C. Beyrer et al. "Safeguarding human health in the Anthropocene epoch: report of the Rockefeller Foundation-*Lancet* Commission on planetary health." *The Lancet*, 16 July 2015, p. 1.

[44]Kenneth Prewitt, personal communication.

[45]Gustav Nossal, personal communication.

character and remained a widely respected, highly talented individual in need of gainful employment. In 1988, two separate events took place simultaneously that had a profound influence on Warren's future. Approaching his 60th birthday, with his enthusiasm for life still intact, Warren's parallel interests in science and literature were about to be utilised in the service of the British press baron, Robert "Bob" Maxwell, described by one of his former editors as "a mercurial man with a monstrous ego."[46] Warren's involvement with the IPPNW, his role in SatelLife, and in the advocacy of electronic publishing had brought him to Maxwell's acquisitive attention. Maxwell was an enormously contentious figure in the economic, social, and political life of Britain for more then half a century. Born into abject poverty in the Carpathian Mountains in Czechoslovakia, Jan Ludvik Hock—as he then was called—succeeded in building a world-wide publishing empire. His orthodox Jewish parents were victims of the Nazis; he escaped and fought with distinction among the ranks of the British Army, eventually attaining the rank of captain. After the end of the Second World War, Ian Robert Maxwell settled in Berlin and using his wartime connections and dynamic self-propulsion became obsessed with scientific publishing. He recognised the historical strength of German institutions in scientific research and development but knew that the social chaos of defeat had diminished this powerful historical status. Nevertheless, some of the infrastructure remained, and he came into contact with the firm of Ferdinand Springer, one of the world's most prestigious scientific publishers. His early dealings with Ferdinand Springer took him all over the world, selling technical publications and reassuring customers that it was morally acceptable to accept such material from a German source. All the time Maxwell recommended the benefits of "pooling scientific data."[47]

Barely six years after making contact with Ferdinand Springer, Maxwell had gone on to co-found the company Lange, Maxwell and Springer (LMS), which had offices in New York City. Maxwell was an enthusiastic Anglophile and spoke with genuine affection for Winston Churchill, whose defiant speeches he listened to on the BBC while fighting fascism in occupied Europe. He founded Pergamon Press in 1949, and the UK was the heartbeat of his publishing empire, which he ran from his palatial home-cum-headquarters in Headington Hill Hall, Oxford. Politically, he espoused left-wing views and served as a Member of Parliament (MP) for the Labour Party from 1964 until 1970. However, even when an MP, the probity of his business dealings began to be questioned by government agencies. After one of his

---

[46]R. Greenslade, "Pension plunderer Robert Maxwell remembered 20 years after his death," *The Guardian*, 3 November 2011.

[47]R. Davies, *Foreign Body: The Secret Life of Robert Maxwell*, Bloomsbury, 1995, p. 168.

more questionable take-over bids, a Department of Trade and Industry report stated, "We regret having to conclude that, notwithstanding Mr. Maxwell's acknowledged abilities and energy, he is not in our opinion a person who can be relied upon to exercise proper stewardship of a publicly quoted company."[48] By this time however, Maxwell was an extremely powerful man: He owned national newspapers; he was friends with leading politicians, particularly in the Communist bloc; and he silenced many of his critics via an insatiable appetite for litigation in the libel courts. One of Maxwell's biographers, Russell Davies, noted a telling feature of the press baron's behaviour: "It was always a habit of Robert Maxwell's to take an interest in the outcast: to move toward his isolation and make him an offer."[49]

In 1988, Maxwell purchased the American publishing firm Macmillan Inc., for \$2.6 billion, and immediately looked for someone with a love of literature and knowledge of modern biomedical science to help run his new acquisition. He set his sights on Warren. Sylvia remembers a meeting of the two men in Oxford: "We went to a party in Oxford and Maxwell arrived in a helicopter. All the other guests were standing around and he came straight over to Ken and ignored everyone else. It was about this time that it was decided, given Ken's interest and knowledge of literature, that he should assist Kevin, Maxwell's youngest son, who was to run Macmillan, in New York. The rest is history."[50] During the meeting, the common ideals of both men were readily evident: Both were fascinated with the idea of electronic information. Warren was convinced that everything should be digitised, and whenever possible, he lobbied journal editors to digitise their material, advocating that the future of medical information would be on computer screens and thus easily accessible to all. Again Warren was a visionary, an outlier for the concept of open access. Maxwell also saw digitisation as the future for his industrial base and discussed how Warren might invent ways to make science profitable and accessible.[51] Building on the political contacts he had cultivated in Eastern Europe, his hope was to make the previously untapped reservoir of Soviet scientific knowledge commercially available in the West. For Warren, linking up with Maxwell was definitely a turn away from the GND focus, but it wasn't out of step with his interests: knowledge transference, integration of scientific and medical publishing,

[48]R. Greenslade, *Maxwell: The Rise and Fall of Robert Maxwell and his empire,* Carol Publishing Group, New York, 1992, p. 36. 'Maxwellisation' is a procedure in British governance where individuals due to be criticised in an official report are sent details of the criticism in advance and permitted to respond prior to publication. The process took its name from Maxwell who took the DTI to court in 1969, with the judge ruling that the DTI criticism had "virtually committed the business murder" of Maxwell.

[49]R. Davies, *Foreign Body: The Secret Life of Robert Maxwell,* Bloomsbury, 1995, p. 30.

[50]Sylvia Warren, personal communication.

[51]Don Bundy, personal communication.

online databases, document delivery, and a close proximity to power.[52] Warren's friend, the epidemiologist Richard Peto, saw the alliance as somewhat prophetic: "I always thought of Ken being a bit like the Robert Maxwell of disease control."[53] Both men were grandiose, larger-than-life figures, and both were viewed with suspicion by the establishment. Warren's annual salary of $225,000 was a vast increase on any previous remuneration that he had received. In addition, his contract also included additional payments of $1200 for his membership of The Century Association, $1000 annual dues to The Harvard Club, a further $600 annual dues to The St. Botolph Club in Boston, and approximately $100 annually for his memberships of the American Association of Immunologists, the American College of Physicians, and the American Society of Tropical Medicine.[54]

Together with being on Maxwell's payroll as Director of Science at Macmillan, in 1988 the other serendipitous event in Warren's life was an invitation from Keith McAdam to give the Heath Clark Lectures at the London School of Hygiene and Tropical Medicine.[55] This was the school's highest honour, and McAdam engineered a 3-month fellowship for Warren, during which time he gave a series of lectures and engaged in the intellectual and social life of the Keppel Street institution. This was a tumultuous period at the school as it sought a new dynamic dean to lead it into the era of global health and to reinvigorate its staff and student body with modular teaching and an up-scaled administrative structure. Warren had a great affection for the school, going back to the days of his Diploma in Tropical Medicine and Hygiene in the late 1950s, and he decided to apply for the deanship. The senior management at the School had set up a search committee to find the new dean, which was chaired by Lord Snow, the Minister of Science. McAdam and many of Warren's GND colleagues believed the job would have been ideal for him,[56] but at the last moment, Richard Feacham, another major figure in the world of infectious diseases, threw his hat into the ring. The search committee now had a list of two names from which to select a new dean. Fatefully, the day before the search committee was due to make the final decision, Robert Maxwell

---

[52]In his contract, which began on 1 January 1989, some of Warren's responsibilities included: 'Analysing and assessing existing information and data base systems (including the management of libraries data bases and the storage, retrieval and distribution of information to customers) and implementing recommendations for the purpose of improving the quality of, and providing more efficient access to, information and data thereto throughout the Maxwell group.' 'Initiating, developing and implementing information systems and programmes for the Maxwell Group to enable customers world-wide to access and utilise efficiently, high-quality information data.' 'Recommending acquisition and participating in the acquisition of relevant journals, books, technologies and companies to achieve overall goals.' 'Otherwise consulting with, advising and assisting management where Dr Warren's knowledge and experience may provide special insight or expertise'.

[53]Sir Richard Peto, personal communication.

[54]Warren's Macmillan contract. Courtesy of Sylvia Warren.

[55]K. S. Warren, "Tropical Medicine or Tropical Health: The Heath Clark Lectures, 1988." Reviews of Infectious Diseases. Vol. 12, No. 1, January-February 1990, pp. 142–155.

[56]Keith McAdam, personal communication.

phoned Lord Snow informing him firstly of what an impressive person Warren was, and secondly that he intended to make a large bequest to the school to upgrade their library and information services.[57] Lord Snow obviously felt Maxwell's blatant approach was inappropriate. Keith McAdam, sitting on the search committee, recalls the effect the conversation had upon Lord Snow: "He said, 'as far as I'm concerned that is the end of the search.' Ken didn't get the job, he was out, and of course, Richard Feachem went on to be a brilliant dean."[58]

Far from ending Maxwell and Warren's relationship, the rejection merely acted to further galvanise it. Maxwell, as observed by Sylvia Warren, "had a tremendous admiration for Ken and what he had achieved."[59] A genuine friendship developed, with Maxwell recognising that he could rely on Warren to provide truthful views and advice. Robert Maxwell had gained a foothold in the world of publishing by way of science and its growing application in the decades after WWII. The reason Maxwell was initially interested in securing the services of Warren was his confidence that there existed a vast resource of scientific information and data in the Soviet Union that could be liberated in a profitable way and utilised in the West. Warren appeared to be a perfect synergistic fit in that he both had contacts in the Soviet Union as well as an interest in scientific publishing. However, after many visits to the Soviet Union, Warren realised that the digital promised-land that Maxwell hoped to exploit did not exist; as a consequence his advice to Maxwell was, "don't get involved."[60]

The total implosion of Maxwell's empire was not yet apparent, and Warren still hoped to persuade Maxwell to fund many of his new ideas for medical publishing together with the planned expansion of the SatelLife programme.[61] Yet, as at the RF, Warren's ambitions with Maxwell were to be cut short. Before Maxwell's death in 1991—he drowned under mysterious circumstances when his luxurious yacht *Lady Ghislaine* was cruising off the coast of the Canary Islands—the British public was content with its idea of Maxwell as a merely local tyrant[62]; Someone who had spent a lifetime gorging, boa-constrictor like, on the excesses of dishonesty, bullying, and gastronomic consumption. For those who witnessed it, who could forget Maxwell in his role as owner of the victorious Oxford United football team, lumbering grotesquely across the pitch of Wembley Stadium to celebrate his team's success in the 1986 Milk Cup Final. His presence, already a source of deep embarrassment to the loyal Oxford United fans, only intensified, when at the post-match interview, Maxwell was unable to remember the name of the club captain, Malcolm Shotton! In the immediate period following Maxwell's death, the misplaced eulogies came to an abrupt end as the full extent of his venality was

---

[57]Sylvia Warren, personal communication.

[58]Keith McAdam, personal communication.

[59]Sylvia Warren, personal communication.

[60]Sylvia Warren, personal communication.

[61]Charlie Clements, personal communication.

[62]R. Davies, *Foreign Body: The Secret Life of Robert Maxwell,* Bloomsbury, 1995, p. 2.

revealed. He had become so desperate for funds that he had stolen some $700 million from his employees' pension funds to keep his companies afloat. Warren's association with Maxwell was, according to Sylvia Warren, "brief and cordial."[63] Warren was one of the more fortunate people who was shown respect by Maxwell, which did not happen to many members of his staff, and certainly not to Peter Jay, a former British Ambassador to the United States and Maxwell's chief of staff during the years of tumult. Sylvia believes that Ken was "perplexed by the accusations levelled at Maxwell and was thankful for the respect and kindness with which he had been treated."[64] Ultimately, far from being a saviour, Maxwell became the poster boy for corruption, forcing Warren once again to seek new patronage to pursue his life in science.

He did not have to wait long. In 1992, Warren's friend, Tony Cerami, invited him to become Vice President for Academic Affairs at the newly constituted Picower Institute for Medical Research in Manhasset on Long Island. Cerami and Warren had first met in 1977 when they were introduced by Jim Hirsch, dean of the Rockefeller University, where Cerami was Professor and Head of the Laboratory of Medical Biochemistry. Warren intended to recruit him into the GND network, and made the then 37-year-old scientist a proposition that he couldn't refuse. Cerami recalls that Warren "offered funding of $100,000 a year for a 10-year period—a remarkable offer. Although I had not studied parasites, I always had an interest in the area since I had first read about Paul Ehrlich in Paul de Kruif's *Microbe Hunters*. Over the next ten years, my laboratory worked on trypanosomiasis, malaria, hookworm and the cachexia associated with infections."[65] This work on cachectic catabolic wasting had a formative influence on Cerami and his standing as a research scientist. In 1981, he wrote a patent that has become a defining blueprint of anti-tumour necrosis- factor therapies, which today is a $20 billion-a-year industry. Like Ehrlich, Cerami was a scientific gambler; then again so too were a great many of the earlier microbe hunters, but he also had scientific intuition and a single-mindedness to discover the mechanisms of disease.

With this in mind, while there undoubtedly was a great bond of personal friendship between Warren and Cerami: The latter also recognised that without the GND he would not have made his breakthrough discovery. Moreover, he also believed that Warren had been treated unfairly by the RF and that the Picower Institute would offer his friend and colleague an opportunity to flourish.

With Jeffry M. Picower's economic support, Cerami had secured $10 million in initial funding from the Florida-based investor for his biomedical research, which was to be guided by a signally benevolent aim: To "find cures for the maladies that afflict humankind."[66] As the President of the new Picower Institute for Medical

---

[63]Sylvia Warren, personal communication.

[64]Sylvia Warren, personal communication.

[65]A. Cerami, "A Surprising Journey in Translational Medicine." *Molecular Medicine,* Vol. 20, (Supplement 1) pp. S2-S6, 2014.

[66]M. Jacoby, *St Petersburg Times* (Florida), 8 July 2001.

Research, Cerami was at the peak of his career, but the new role had come at some considerable personal cost. Cerami had been embroiled in an internecine power struggle with Dr. David Baltimore, the distinguished scientist and Nobel laureate. Cerami opposed Baltimore's appointment as president of Rockefeller University on the grounds that he had been connected with a case of scientific misconduct. In an article written on 1 August 1991, the *New York Times* journalist William K. Stevens explained the background to the disagreement, revealing that "a special investigative panel of the National Institute of Health found earlier this year that a former associate of Dr. Baltimore, Dr. Thereza Imanishi-Kari, had faked data in a 1986 research paper. The challenged research was not done at Dr. Baltimore's laboratory, but he signed the paper as a co-author while he headed the Whitehead Institute in Cambridge, Massachusetts. He consistently defended his associate but apologised for the prolonged defense after the investigative panel made its finding. Dr. Cerami, in opposing Dr. Baltimore's appointment at Rockefeller in 1989, said that his handling of the case 'got him in more trouble than if he had handled it in a straightforward manner from the beginning' and that this had become 'a bellwether for his character.'"

The situation proved untenable, and although Baltimore's presidency was certainly ill-fated, lasting a mere 18 months, nonetheless, Cerami took the decision to relocate to the Picower Institute, taking his entire 30-strong research team—and Ken Warren—with him. One of Warren's many tasks was to oversee the running of the MD–PhD programme (now known as the Elmezzi Graduate School). Also, from the laboratories at the Picower Institute, Warren continued his research into the subject that had been his life-long fascination: helminth infection. The worm that held particular fascination for him was *Ascaris lumbricoides*, the big roundworm.[67] From his work with Julia Walsh on selective primary health care, Warren emphasised the need for science, measurement, data, and reasoned analysis, and he recognised that any treatment needed to be cost-effective: low in cost but high in impact. In many ways, helminths were the prototypical great neglected disease with hookworm, ascariasis, trichuriasis, and enterobiasis combining to produce more than 3 billion infections globally. This quest to understand the ecology of infection brought the work of the British epidemiologist Donald Bundy to his attention. Warren was captivated by the work Bundy was doing on the population dynamics of the ascaris worm. Bundy's research built upon the ideas developed by the epidemiologist Roy Anderson and the theoretical ecologist Bob May, which stated that if it were possible to take the intensity of parasitism below some threshold in a given village, and to keep it low, that it was possible to drive the parasite to local extinction.[68] The possibility of recording the burden of infection, the number of worms that people were infected with, the pattern of infection, and how that might influence treatment, was something that had not yet been considered by

---

[67]N. R. Stoll, "This Wormy World," Journal of Parasitology, 33: 1–18, 1947.

[68]W. G. Esch, *Parasites and Infectious Disease: Discovery by Serendipity and Otherwise.* Cambridge University Press, 2007, p. 40.

parasitologists and epidemiologists. Here Bundy explains the philosophy under-pinning the hypothesis: "It was the realisation that you could think about these worms as though they were really animals, like rabbits in a field, in occupying us, not like the viruses, or the bacteria or the protozoa, where the question would be 'how many people are infected?' The number of people infected determines who else is going to be infected. You are following the trajectory of infection from individual to individual host, whereas with these worms, the number of worms determines how infectious the person was. The more worms, the more eggs. This made all the difference to thinking about the epidemiology, because what then matters is not now many people you treat, or how many people you vaccinate, which of course is true for most of the diseases we're thinking of, it is actually how many worms you get rid of."[69] Bundy's observation revealed that if one person in a hundred had a thousand worms, treating that one person would have a big impact on how to design control programmes. Indeed, given that school children had a greater burden of worms than any other group, his work led to the recognition that by focusing treatment on schools, it would be possible to remove 70% of the worms in the whole population and thus reduce the level of infection transmission.

Warren was immediately attracted to the policy implications of Bundy's work, and when Seth Berkley organised a meeting on the Health of School-Age Children at Bellagio in August 1991, Warren and Bundy were attendees.[70] They followed this up with a multi-authored paper in 1993 that appeared as a chapter in the highly influential publication *Disease Control Priorities* and which was also a background paper informing *The World Development Report: Investing in Health*.[71] The paper compiled a whole set of arguments based on the new parasite ecology/epidemiology work and highlighted for the first time that relatively innocuous helminth infections actually had insidious effects, affecting cognitive and other development, and that this realisation could change contemporary visions of the burden of disease. Don Bundy recalls that the work "caused a furor in the business, because suddenly these unimportant great neglected worms had disability consequences far greater than some of these more common diseases, and that caused a good deal of rethinking at the time, and it has had its legacy. Ken loved that. That was exactly what he had been saying, that there is this huge level of infection and that it has consequences. Today we know that now to be true."[72] The epidemiological approach of using scientifically designed chemotherapy programmes is what now defines the Neglected Tropical Diseases movement, and the inclusion of cognitive development as a "health" outcome was an early push toward the burden-of-disease approach. Even late in his career, Warren continued to help push the boundaries of science.

[69]Don Bundy, personal communication.

[70]K. S. Warren, "Helminths and health of school-age children." *The Lancet*, Vol. 338, 14 Sept 1991, pp. 686–687.

[71]K. S. Warren, D. A. P. Bundy, R. M. Anderson, A. R. Davies, D. A. Anderson, D. T. Jamison, N. Prescott & A. Senft, "Helminth Infection", in D. T. Jamison, W. H. Mosley, A. R. Measham & J. L. Bobadilla (eds), *Disease Control Priorities*, Oxford University Press, 1993, pp. 131–160.

[72]Don Bundy, personal communication.

An undeniable feature of Warren's life was its extraordinary diversity; while agitating for programmes of chemotherapy and prophylaxis, he also campaigned for greater analysis and systematic reviews of health-care interventions, building on his earlier work on the metrics of biomedical literature. In 1993, he spoke at length on the topic at the New York Academy of Sciences meeting, a gathering that had been orchestrated around the theme of "Doing More Good than Harm: The Evaluation of Health Care Interventions."

The shift of emphasis toward a more critical evaluation of health interventions was made still more apparent by the establishment, in the same year, of The Cochrane Collaboration in Oxford. As the eponymous Archie Cochrane had lamented, "it is surely a great criticism of our profession that we have not organised a critical summary, by specialty or subspecialty, adapted periodically, of all relevant randomised controlled trials (RCTs)."[73] The new organisation was the brainchild of Iain Chalmers and was founded as a non-profit body that would systematically organise research information. Now rolled out across the globe, the Cochrane Collaboration has a presence in 100 countries with more then 28,000 volunteers contributing to its dedicated aim of making the latest, accurate information about the effects of health care readily available worldwide. In recognition of Warren's early encouragement and interest, particularly in tropical diseases, it was decided after Warren's death in 1996 to establish the Kenneth Warren Prize as a memorial to him within the Cochrane Collaboration.

This was a period of considerable cross-pollination of ideas for Warren, borne out of his friendship with, and admiration for, the work of Chalmers and Richard Peto. Chalmers had produced the first medical textbook based on RCTs and meta-analysis,[74] whereas Peto had developed large-scale,[75] multi-center randomised controlled trials for the study of chronic diseases[76] and developed statistical methods for combining RCTs by way of meta-analysis. Through his own work in medical information science and international clinical epidemiology, Warren became closely involved with both Peto and Chalmers. Particularly during the period when working for Maxwell, he would often be in Oxford looking for ways to collaborate in the production of an electronic database of RCTs and meta-analyses that would specifically answer physicians' clinical enquiries. One of Chalmers' collaborators in Oxford during this period was the publishing entrepreneur Mark Starr, who saw that Warren had similar thoughts about how to get scientific information to make a difference: "What I liked about Ken was that firstly, he was enthusiastic, he'd listen to any idea whether it was about schistosomiasis or electronic publishing. I was on the electronic publishing side of this whole thing, and

---

[73]The Cochrane Centre (brochure). National Health Service Research and Development Programme. Oxford, 1992.

[74]I. Chalmers, M. Enkin & M. J. N. Keirse, *A Guide to Effective Care in Pregnancy and Childbirth*, Oxford University Press, 1989.

[75]R. Peto, "Clinical trial methodology." *Biomedicine* 1978, 28 (special issue): 24–36.

[76]C. Keating, "The social history of ISIS-2: the early history." *The Lancet*, 2015, 386, 646–647.

what I liked about him was that he was one of those people who 'got it.' He understood Cochrane, the idea of systematic reviews that would be regularly updated, and he understood the idea of electronic publishing, the move forward into an electronic world ... he was our big hope for funding."[77]

In 1993, Warren didn't have access to the financial resources he once did, but his own work in epidemiology, largely in the developing world, taught him the importance of medical economics and the setting of priorities for health care initiatives in financially constrained parts of the world.[78] He amalgamated faultlessly a dedication to library networks in developing countries and the mathematical analysis of medical literature and championed the use of randomised controlled trials to improve all human health. By participating in the New York Academy of Sciences meeting of 1993 (Doing More Good Than Harm) and editing the conference proceedings, he helped contribute to the gestation of "valuable suggestions" about how "new knowledge could be transmitted to medical practitioners." ensuring in the words of the conference summation, given by Sir Richard Doll, that the meeting might mark "a turning point in the history of medicine in the developed world."[79]

Another major contribution to information sciences came in 1994, when Warren co-founded the journal *Molecular Medicine*, a joint publication of the Picower Institute Press and Blackwell Science, Inc., which became the official journal of the Molecular Medicine Society. With Cerami as editor-in-chief and Warren as deputy-editor, the journal's aims were to serve as a platform for the greater understanding of the mechanisms of disease, to signpost the way forward for physician–scientists to develop treatments for common diseases, and to champion translational medicine by linking research in the laboratory to treatment in the clinic. Meanwhile, Warren's dedication to systematic reviews and speeding up access to medical discoveries had brought him into contact with Vitek Tracz, the London-based publishing entrepreneur. Tracz was an innovator, a pioneer of the open-access movement that transfigured medical publishing at the end of the twentieth century, who was once described by Richard Smith (former editor of the *British Medical Journal*) as "the Picasso of science publishing" not only because of a physical similarity to the artist but also for the striking originality of how he envisioned and shaped the publishing world. Tracz, Chalmers, Starr, and

[77]Mark Starr, personal communication.

[78]J. A. Walsh & K. S. Warren, "Selective primary health care: An interim strategy for disease control in developing countries." N. Engl. J. Med, 1979, 301: 967–974.

[79]R. Doll, 1993. "Summation of the conference," in K. S. Warren & F. Mosteller (eds), *Doing More Good than Harm: The Evaluation of Interventions*, Annals of the New York Academy of Sciences 703, 1993, pp. 310–313.

Warren occupied the same intellectual scientific biosphere; all were dedicated to open access, systematic reviews, and providing the most up-to-date medical information to the greatest number at the lowest cost.

Indeed, Warren was ahead of most health professionals in investing in the capacity to collect large amounts of accurate data and make it available to many. Through the programmes he developed at the RF and subsequently, he ensured that there was an increase in capacity all over the world in accurate data collection for disease surveillance and epidemiology and a greater availability of information and recent publications for all. Furthermore, he remained strong in his belief that having current science journal articles available in all libraries around the world was essential for nurturing and stimulating scientists from developing countries. These multifarious achievements in the development of information science shaped the future that we now inhabit. Warren's quest for low-cost subscriptions to journals, access to scientific databases, and search algorithms that could accurately select relevant articles together formed a powerful influence in the historical trajectory of the discipline. In the words of Julia Walsh, "these priorities align with, and presaged by a decade or more, the current efforts for Open Access journals, better cataloging and searching for peer-reviewed and grey literature, and big data for better surveillance and knowledge about new trends in disease and outbreaks."[80]

Ken Warren still had ideas, and just as importantly, the influence and energy to fulfill their potential: He still had sovereignty over his destiny. Yet on one occasion in the mid-1990s, Vitek Tracz visited his friend at the Picower Institute for Medical Research and made a telling observation: "I went to see him on Long Island. It didn't seem right to me. He was a little lost."[81] Conceivably Tracz registered the diminishment in power, vision, and the eclipsing of the once seemingly irreducible energy that Warren had exuded. Warren may have begun to realise that his years at the RF were going to be the high water mark of his career. After all, he had given his labor, service, and humanity to some of the forgotten people of the world; now on Long Island, he may have revealed unconsciously that he knew he would never make such a contribution again. In one sense, Ken Warren had been unlucky: His main post-Rockefeller employers were venal individuals who lacked moral integrity. The Jeffry Picower financial empire, a toxic nexus of wealth, power, and deceit, would implode causing even greater collateral damage than the downfall of Robert Maxwell. But by then Ken Warren would no longer be alive.

---

[80]Julia Walsh, personal communication.

[81]Vitek Tracz, personal communication.

Chapter 6
Warren in Retrospect

Harvard played a formative role in shaping Ken Warren because it was there that his joint passions for literature and medicine became co-equal and co-eternal in his life. At Harvard College, he devoted his time to literature, poetry, and the works of William Shakespeare. Later, at Harvard Medical School, he embraced the spirit of his chosen profession, healing the sick. There, too, he became a member of the celebrated Aesculapian Club, which was established in 1902 by Townsend W. Throndike, a fourth-year medical student who organised his classmates into a society, "which would undertake work for the interests of the School." The club seal is a circle formed by the Aesculapian Serpent with the motto from Ambroise Paré, "We dress the wound; God heals it." Renowned for its sense of camaraderie, the club was where he cultivated a taste for smoking cigars, drinking malt whisky, and fine dining. "It was," remembered Sylvia Warren, "a good living group when Ken was there."[1] As a consequence of this enduring connection, it was unsurprising that when the Dana-Farber Cancer Institute (a principal teaching affiliate of Harvard Medical School) began an epidemiological study looking at survival rates among former cancer patients, Warren, who in his 40s had has melanoma, joined the cohort. It was the early summer of 1996, and the blood still pounded along his veins; he felt healthy, perhaps because for 20 years he had assiduously self administered the BCG vaccine.

Warren believed that the medical profession had a responsibility not only for the cure of the sick and for the prevention of disease but also for the advancement of knowledge on which both depend. He was interested in epidemiology, meta-analysis, large-scale randomised evidence, and large-scale implementation. Indeed, one of his reasons for entering the Harvard study was the hope that his participation would produce some reliable evidence for future generations. Yet Warren's presence in the cohort also had profoundly personal ramifications. At one of his routine visits to the Dana-Farber Cancer Institute, it was discovered that he had metastatic disease; a tumour was found in his brain, and the prognosis was that he only had a few months to live.

---

[1]Sylvia Warren, personal communication.

© Springer International Publishing AG 2017
C. Keating, *Kenneth Warren and the Great Neglected Diseases
of Mankind Programme*, Springer Biographies,
DOI 10.1007/978-3-319-50147-5_6

Warren knew that his destiny was now defined by the natural development of the disease, but he refused to change his way of life.[2] He still bustled with the other commuters on the long train journey from Dobbs Ferry to The Picower Institute for Research on Long Island. It was there on June 19th that a great gathering of his friends and collaborators came to celebrate his contribution to medical science. Dressed in the graduation robes of Mahidol University, Bangkok, whose Department of Biochemistry had been an integral part of the original GND network, Warren accepted an honorary degree—the first ever presented at the Picower Institute—as well as the accolades, speeches of kind recognition, and diverting humour from the guests assembled from across the world. John Bruer spoke with light-hearted and good natured comments. It was the last time that he would see Ken Warren alive.[3] John David acknowledged that, other than his family, no one had changed his life more than Ken Warren. When he spoke, he was unambiguous about the debt that he owed: "There is no question, what I have done, going into parasitology, starting the Woods Hole course, ending up being Chairman of the Department of Public Health, all of that would never have happened without Ken Warren (Fig. 6.1)."[4]

Looking already noticeably debilitated, Warren used the degree ceremony to thank his friend, "my alter ego Tony Cerami," for his support and scientific perspicacity.[5] He also paid this tribute to his family: "To my remarkable wife and the two idealistic children whom she nurtured, who both care deeply for those who need help in this world. They not only had to put up with lightning striking all over the place, but with the rigors of an underpaid academic career with no advanced clinical training and no income whatsoever from patients, with intense scientific ambition which means, as so many of you know, six to seven day weeks, ten to twelve hour days. In addition, there were the many periods of travel throughout the world required by a career in tropical medicine, and the longer periods when the whole family were dragged off to Brazil, St Lucia, Kenya and Egypt. Moreover I always believed that I had to fulfill my destiny driven by science and helping my fellow human beings wherever it provided the best opportunity. Your life has not been easy. For that I apologise. I hope that at least it has been interesting."[6] Such heartfelt gratitude was all the more unforeseen because Ken Warren could not be described as a family man. Warren's dedication to geographic and tropical medicine and to helping the world's poorest people came at a cost. Conceivably Sylvia's own family background helped nurture a forbearance for the considerable burden she was to bear. As she recalls, "we were all tearful, because it was so unexpected. We definitely came second; Ken's work was his priority. He was not involved with the kids, even when we did go with him abroad, he was working all day, and frequently

---

[2]Sylvia Warren, personal communication.

[3]John Bruer, personal communication.

[4]John David, personal communication.

[5]K. S. Warren, Speech given 19 June 1996. Courtesy of Sylvia Warren.

[6]K. S. Warren, Speech given 19 June 1996. Courtesy of Sylvia Warren.

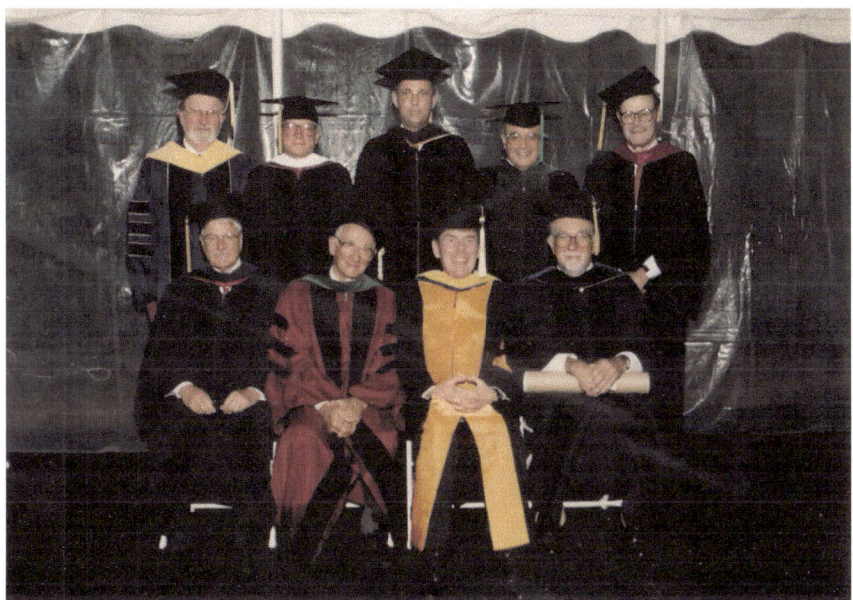

Fig. 6.1 Group Photograph Honorary Degree taken at the Picower Institute of Medical Research June 19, 1996. *Left to right, top row* Jere Goyan (former dean of UCSF and former commissioner of the FDA, *third from left*, John Bruer, *fourth from left*, Adel Mahmoud, and David Nathan, Harvard Medical School. *Left to right, bottom row* C Leonard Gordon, former classmate and roommate of Ken Warren's at Harvard College. John David, former Head of Parasitology at Harvard Medical School, Ken Warren and Tony Cerami. Courtesy of Sylvia Warren

in the evening. It was the same with my father; his science came first. I grew up with an absolute workaholic (Fig. 6.2)."[7]

Since the late 1980s, Ken and Sylvia had been ploughing their savings into restoring Rysted, the resplendent art-deco house that Sylvia's father had built in the 1930s. Set in rolling hills outside the village of Westerham in Kent, England, it seemed the ideal location for a productive retirement. Warren had built a spacious wooden chalet, which he called his "communications centre," at the bottom of the vertiginous garden where he had planned to oversee the transmission of health information to the developing world. The communications centre's hub was a desk that Onesmo ole-MoiYoi had sent from Kenya as a gift to the friend who had inspired his research work at the International Laboratory for Research on Animal Diseases.[8] Warren was a great Anglophile, and the bucolic Kent countryside made for a perfect site, especially because Rysted was where Sylvia's peripatetic heart had always longed to settle. By the summer of 1996, the restoration was complete; the Crittall steel-framed corner windows gave the house an authenticity that it had

---

[7]Sylvia Warren, personal communication.

[8]Letter from O. K. Ole-MoiYoi to K. S. Warren, 19 May 1993. Courtesy of Sylvia Warren.

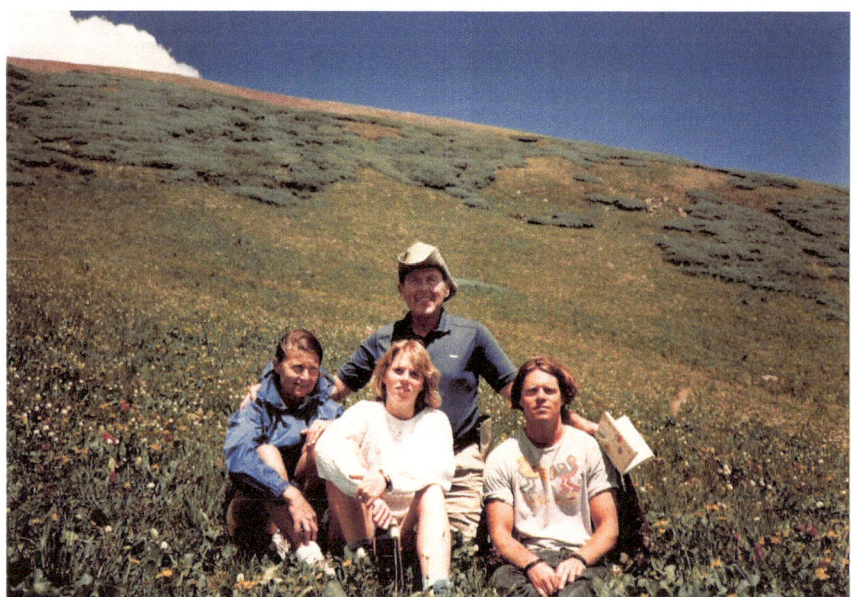

Fig. 6.2 The Warren family on holiday in Colorado for Ken and Sylvia's joint 60th birthdays. Courtesy of Erica Warren

not possessed for a generation. The flat-roofed house still presents a glittering luminescence; with its brilliant white walls and Mediterranean blue and silver paintwork, one is reminded of a stream-lined ocean vessel from the 1930s.

Although it was now impossible to camouflage his failing health, Warren was determined to visit Rysted for one last time, to sit in his communications centre, and to catch up with like-minded friends and colleagues in the UK. Exhausted by his illness, Warren was losing his mobility, and he needed the use of a wheelchair when he accompanied Sylvia to an exhibition in London as part of her birthday celebrations on 22 July 1996. Of course, there was still time for work. During that golden summer of 1996, three major figures in British epidemiology visited him at Rysted. Richard Peto, Don Bundy, and Iain Chalmers drove down from Oxford and had lunch with him and Sylvia. All of the epidemiologists had been influenced, funded, inspired, or helped in their work in some way by Warren, and they wanted to see him and discuss ideas. Iain Chalmers remembers that "Ken was very frail by that time, and Richard Peto spoke about a proposed randomised trial and said that they would dedicate the report to him.[9]

The speed of Warren's decline accelerated to such a degree that Tony Cerami came over from the US and paid for the first-class transit of Ken and Sylvia back to

---

[9]S. Awasthi et al. "Population deworming every 6 months with albendazole in 1 million pre-school children in north India. DEVTA, a cluster-randomised trial." *The Lancet*, 2013, 381: 1478–86.

New York. The news that Ken Warren was approaching the end of his life spread rapidly through the global health community. The tragic news arrived at a telling moment for Dick Guerrant in Charlottesville, Virginia: "I phoned his home and told him that I had publicly thanked him in the acknowledgements of a book we had just published with colleagues in northeastern Brazil.[10] I said, 'I just want you to know that our work in Brazil, *you made it possible*, and I just want to personally say thank you and that I know that you've had some crummy news recently.' And his response was, 'Don't feel sorry for me Dick; I've just had the most fantastic twenty years of great life, that I wasn't supposed to have.' And I was just blown away. Would that we could all appreciate and celebrate life like Ken!."[11] Now near the end of his life, Warren wrote to his friend, Richard Peto.[12] Among his positive ruminations on life, the letter contained the final two lines from Shakespeare's "Sonnet 12":

And nothing 'gainst Time's Scythe

Can make defence

Save breed, to brave him when he

takes thee hence

Much of Warren's professional life was dedicated to helminthology and the science of epidemiology, which he described unsentimentally as being "compassion with the tears wiped away."[13] Characteristically, even in the last period of his life, he was encouraging of Peto's idea of a randomised trial to help assess the effects of regular deworming on mortality amongst 1 million children in India. In the study by Awasthi et al., which was published in 2013, it seemed only fitting that Warren's memory was celebrated with a quote from Shakespeare: "This report is dedicated to its onlie begetter, Kenneth S. Warren (1929–1996)."[14] Warren could not, to quote the poet Dylan Thomas, "rage against the dying of the light," but he did face death with an enviable equanimity. Kenneth S. Warren, M.D. died from malignant melanoma on 18 September 1996 at his home in Dobbs Ferry. He was 67 years old.

One of the jobs of the historian is to remember what others forget. On 14 May 2015, the science journalist Amy Nordrum wrote an intriguing article entitled "How Three Scientists 'Marketed' Neglected Tropical Diseases And Raised More Than $1 Billion." The article, which appeared in the *International Business Times*, told the story of how David Molyneux, Peter Hotez, and Alan Fenwick had used the

---

[10]R. L. Guerrant, M. Auxiliadoro de Souza & M. K. Nations (eds), *At the Edge of Development: Health Crises in a transitional society*, Durham, N.C., Carolina Academic Press, 1996.

[11]Dick Guerrant, personal communication.

[12]Richard Peto, personal communication.

[13]Richard Peto, personal communication.

[14]S. Awasthi et al. "Population deworming every 6 months with albendazole in 1 million pre-school children in north India. DEVTA, a cluster-randomised trial." *The Lancet*, 2013, 381: 1478–86.

term 'neglected tropical diseases' to create a "surge in funding in the last decade."[15] Money had come from the Bill and Melinda Gates Foundation, from the U.S. Agency for International Development, and from pharmaceutical companies. Nordrum went on to quote Josh Michaud, Associate Director for Global Health at the Kaiser Family Foundation, "Marketing is a big aspect of it," Michaud stated. "Had they not come up with this term, I don't think we would be where we are in terms of funding and attention on this issue." Dorie Clark, a branding expert, was also quoted in the article, saying, "I think the term 'neglected tropical diseases' is a brilliant umbrella term. It allows funders to feel like they are addressing something important that has been hidden for a long time."

What had concentrated the minds of Molyneux, Hotez, and Fenwick was the establishment in 2002 of a new private–public partnership, The Global Fund to Fight AIDS, Tuberculosis and Malaria. This organisation was underpinned by substantial long-term funding, while at the time the diseases to which the researchers had devoted much of their lives—schistosomiasis, hookworm, lymphatic filariasis, and guinea worm—remained neglected and underfunded. Therefore, to attract new funding streams and greater attention to what they believed to be truly neglected tropical diseases, they launched their commendable campaign in 2005, which in effect refashioned NTDs to the world by making something old new again.

Ken Warren's contribution was not entirely sidelined in Nordrum's telling of the story because the article recorded that "back in the 1970s and 1980s, a researcher named Ken Warren at the Rockefeller Foundation had led an effort to address the world's 'Great Neglected Diseases' which included malaria and schistosomiasis, but that legacy has slowly faded." With the passing of time, Warren's legacy was being obscured by an invisible wall of historical amnesia.

It is true that many people today working in the field of global health will have never heard of Ken Warren. This can partly be understood by the realisation that we live in an ahistorical world. School students may well have heard of Edward Jenner, and medical students might know about the work of Richard Doll, Richard Peto, Selman Waksman, or Philip Hench, but we live in a time when subjects beyond the territory of a 10-year literature review become far off places about which little is known. Science is developing at an ever-increasing pace in which the work of past decades is rapidly superseded. Indeed, most biomedical scientists will be forgotten as the future's enticing potential becomes ever more the focus for new generations of physician–scientists. Is it unsurprising then that with the passing of time, Warren's contribution occupies a curious status in space and time? Although his achievements still reverberate down the decades, they are strangely orphaned from their progenitor. His legacy has not been entirely eclipsed, but there is still no full critical appraisal of his work or, until now, a full-length biography.

---

[15]A. Nordrum, "How Three Scientists 'Marketed' Neglected Tropical Diseases And Raised More Than $1 Billion," *International Business Times*, New York, 14 May 2015.

Now 20 years after his death, as the chain of memory becomes broken, Warren's contribution to medical science is in danger of being neglected, but his attitude, the zeal for the life scientific, and his refusal to take "no" for an answer remain the guiding principles for many who want to help improve the lives of the poor in the developing world. Although Warren did not discover a life-enhancing vaccine, he had a huge influence on the ways in which scientists, administrators, politicians, and funders approached both disease control and the developing world as a whole. Researchers now look at neglected tropical diseases in a more robust way and focus increasingly on morbidity as well as mortality.[16] With this in mind, in writing this book, I aim not to re-direct the story of neglected tropical diseases but to reinstate a man without whom this history cannot be complete.

Of course, it can be argued that compared with other directors of the RF at the time, or with his leading contemporaries in health philanthropy—people of the stature of Joe Cook and Bridget Ogilvie—Warren "is remembered better than most."[17] Certainly any foundation executive who achieves recognition above and beyond their job is quite exceptional. When first hired by the RF, Warren was encouraged by John Knowles to celebrate the traditions of the activist scholar, recognising that while he was primarily working in an administrative role it was incumbent on him to remain active, in an understandably reduced way, in his field of scholarship. And Warren certainly did that; Julia Walsh started her collaborative work with Warren in 1978 and recognised his efforts to reconcile these two imperatives: "Ken was full of more energy and enthusiasm than any other scientist or academic I had worked with previously. Working with him frequently felt like an effort to keep up. An example of his energy and productivity was the research collaborations he maintained at Case Western medical school while he worked non-stop at the RF, designing and implementing several large RF programmes such as the Great Neglected Diseases and Information Science."[18] Warren went on to instill this scholarship ideal in his own staff, emphasising the importance of maintaining an identity in the scientific literature, receiving honest criticism, and trying if at all possible to avoid the perils of foundation institutionalisation where all jokes are laughed at, all ideas are lionised, and all telephone calls are promptly returned.

Being an activist scholar perfectly suited Warren's multifarious interests, and the Stakhanovite levels of productivity that he could harness at the coalface of science helped to extend his bibliographical record to the world. His publications in tropical medicine and parasitology, immunology, and scientific-information systems resulted in him being among the 1000 most cited contemporary authors in the Science Citation Index.[19] In fact, given that Warren developed a distinct philosophy

---

[16]Don Bundy, personal communication.

[17]John Bruer, personal communication.

[18]Julia Walsh, personal communication.

[19]K. S. Warren, "All Effective Treatment Could be Free," December 1993.

on the health of the people in the tropics[20] and contributed profoundly to the metamorphosis and global prestige of parasitology while disbursing $100 million during his decade at the RF, the question might be why his contribution has not attracted more recognition? Richard Peto worked with Warren on many health programmes for the developing world, and here constructs a persuasive chain-reaction diagnosis as to why his colleague's status in the history of global health is not more widely acknowledged: "When he [Warren] eventually got fired as Director of Health Sciences, he was replaced by people who very much didn't want to mention any previous research directors, so somehow his name got written out of history… Once one gets fired from something like the Rockefeller … everyone transfers loyalty pretty sharply. I think Ken was a much more influential figure than is generally appreciated. He caused a lot of other people to do things and his questioning caused a lot of people to think more clearly. [But] because he came to things through being head of a funding agency, once you no longer had that power, suddenly you became a non-person. He had all sorts of influences that as soon as he was stripped of his power, nobody spoke of him, a bit like King Lear."[21]

Although Warren deserves to be remembered as a world-leading research scientist in his own right, particularly during his time at Case Western Reserve, his greatest legacy is to be found in his Rockefeller years. Never short of grandiose ideas or audacious undertakings, it was while at the RF that Warren more fully developed his vision for how best to align scientific discovery to the reduction of disease. Coupled with his innate excitement for science, he brought knowledge and creativity to one of the most influential positions in international philanthropy and health. Employing thought that was way ahead of most people's when it came to disease control, Warren's accomplishments were numerous and profound. At root, he contributed to reviving the field of tropical medicine from a colonial discipline into the mainstream of modern medicine. Through the GND programme, he reshaped molecular biology by drawing top scientists to work on new areas of tropical disease in which they may not otherwise have been interested. These scientists formed new and long-lasting partnerships across and between the developed and developing world and themselves went on to foster a cascade of new tropical-medicine specialists who are now at the forefront of research. Beyond the deepening of scientific knowledge and interactions, Warren also profoundly affected the very ways in which research of the future would be performed. As a creative and innovative grant maker, Warren had a rare talent, personifying the ideals of effective philanthropy and rigorous research and, just as importantly, a feel for the ideas and the people that would shape the future. In utilising relatively modest resources—especially by today's standards—and articulating health in terms of investment rather than expenditure, he had a great effect on the course of

---

[20]K. S. Warren, "Tropical Medicine or Tropical Health: The Heath Clark Lectures, 1988." Reviews of Infectious Diseases. Vol. 12, No. 1, January-February 1990.

[21]Sir Richard Peto, personal communication.

research in tropical medicine and profoundly influenced investment and resources allocation at UNICEF, WHO, USAID, and the World Bank.[22]

Warren was always attracted to difficult subjects, and his concentration on neglected tropical diseases, which affected the distant developing world rather than the immediate first world, deserves to be celebrated. Philosophically, the ethos of the Great Neglected Diseases Programme was guided by one humanitarian principle: All lives have an equal value. The recent and devastating outbreak of Ebola, which occurred in three of the world's poorest countries—Guinea, Liberia, and Sierra Leone—generated fears in those living in rich, more-developed countries that the disease could spread to their parts of the world. But in focusing on diseases that could *only* thrive in the tropical world, Warren did not have that card to play; he could talk about the excitement of the science, the care of the poor, and the need to reduce life-long morbidity, but he could not use his constituency, the neglected poor, to generate the self-interested fears among rich countries that would provide the funds for social amelioration.

Instead, rather than using society to mobilise the scientific and financial communities, Warren used his greatest—and at times most self-defeating—asset: his personality. In the language of modern philanthropy, Warren had "convening power," which he used to assemble powerful agencies, people, and institutions on behalf of the poor and the sick. Unashamedly, he exploited the kudos and the pulling power of the Bellagio to attract powerful decision makers. He aspired to immunise the world's poorest children against killer diseases, and he would not take "no" for an answer. However, at the same time he recognised the significance of human agency, the importance of the individual scientist, and the toll that the hard-labour of a life in science could exact. This is perhaps why he emphasised the excitement and the fun of science; that it was alright to be wrong, and that what was important was to enjoy the thrill of the experiment. In return, and with a little luck, the work would in some small way be relevant to the people in need of help. This collective endeavour brings to mind Lewis Thomas's depiction of the life scientific, seen at times as a lonely activity and yet communal and interdependent. If the objective is to find a single piece of truth about nature, the "whole scientific enterprise must be arranged so that the separate imaginations in different human minds can be pooled, and this is more a kind of game than a systematic business. It is in the abrupt, unaccountable aggregation of random notions, intuitions, known in science as good ideas, that the high points are made."[23] Although Warren could be combative with his superiors and perceived competitors, and his autocratic style at times caused resentment, his warmth and encouragement in dealing with collaborators, junior colleagues, and protégés meant that he was an excellent player of Thomas' scientific "game." He was loyal to his grantees, chose people whom he respected, and persuaded them to work on the diseases that *he* wanted them to work

---

[22]Julia Walsh, personal communication.

[23]L. Thomas, "Natural Science," in *The Lives of a Cell; Notes of a Biology Watcher*, New York: Viking Press, 1974, pp. 100–103.

on. This he managed to achieve with a combination of bonhomie, mind-expanding enthusiasm and mutual respect.[24]

Warren's GND programme, acknowledged by some as "one of the greatest initiatives in tropical medicine research that the world has witnessed," brought about a fundamental redirection of the field.[25] Its generous funding provisions allowed new institutions to flourish, partnerships to be set up between the developed and the developing world, and fledgling programmes to become established world leaders that could nurture new generations of scientists. Such a transformation can be traced at the Parasitology Programme at the Walter and Eliza Hall Institute in Melbourne (WEHI). At the time of the initial funding (1978), the WEHI programme, initiated by Gus Nossal and Graham Mitchell, had been in existence for 3 years and had focused on the immunology of parasitism using mouse model systems. Contact had been made with the Papua New Guinea Institute of Medical Research, but malaria research only began to expand rapidly after the GND grant and the recruitment of Robin Anders and Graham Brown. Subsequently, a long-term research programme on schistosomiasis was started with the Institute (later College) of Public Health in Manila and Sorsogon, Philippines, while ground-breaking work on another human parasite, *Leishmania major*, was performed by Emanuela Handman, who arrived as a post-doctoral fellow at WEHI in 1977. Meanwhile, Gus Nossal was instrumental in directing the molecular biologist, David Kemp, toward malaria research. His team developed a method for screening expression libraries with antibodies used to isolate *Plasmodium falciparum* genes that were potential candidates for vaccine development. Kemp later embarked on new studies looking at ways to alleviate the impact of scabies, the contagious skin infection, which affected many aboriginal Australians.[26] Thus the GND programme enabled WEHI to shift its focus from immunological studies of parasitic diseases in mouse models to studies of human parasites, molecular approaches, and strong linkages with disease-endemic countries in the region (Fig. 6.3).[27]

As Nossal notes, "the new generation of scientists that Ken got involved in this world-wide tidal wave of research" continued to be funded even after Warren left the Rockefeller, an outcome that perfectly suited Warren's aspiration to leave behind something that could be sustained without either him or the RF.[28] Indeed, Warren orchestrated an ingenious financial continuity for WEHI as he handled his own enforced exit strategy. This achievement greatly impressed Gus Nossal, then Director of WEHI: "We received ten wonderful years of support from Ken, and then the time came when the Rockefeller had to change its direction, but he advised the very rich, but not yet experienced, McArthur Foundation to pick up where he

---

[24]Keith McAdam, personal communication.

[25]K. S. Warren & C. C. Jimenez (eds), *The Great Neglected Diseases of Mankind Biomedical Research Network: 1978–1988*. New York: The Rockefeller Foundation, 1988, p. 49.

[26]Louis H. Miller, personal communication.

[27]Graham Mitchell, personal communication.

[28]Gus Nossal, personal communication.

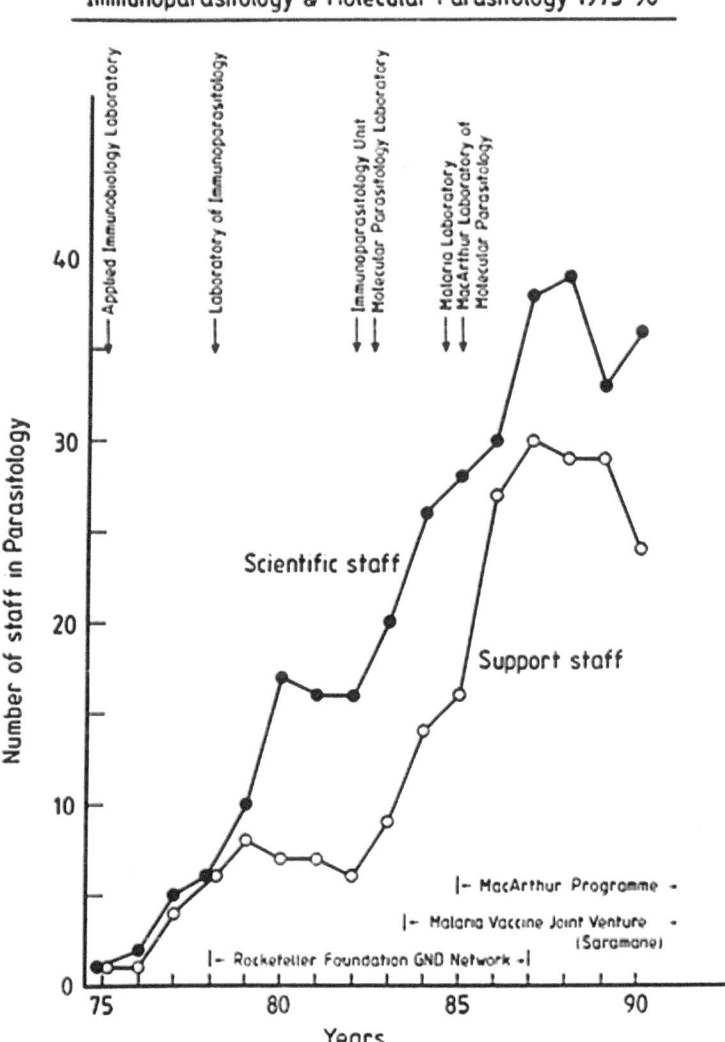

Fig. 6.3 This graph demonstrates the growth of the Parasitology programme at the Walter and Eliza Hall Institute of Medical Research, which, in large part, was funded by the GND research network. Courtesy of Graham Mitchell

left off. And the MacArthur Foundation entered this field and gave us, and doubtless many others, very considerable grant support after the Rockefeller left the field. So, in a way, the ten-year GND gift became a twenty-year gift."[29] The

---

[29]Gus Nossal, personal communication.

McArthur grant enabled parasite molecular biology to become a dominant theme in the quest for molecular vaccines, studies on the intricacies of host-parasite relationships, and the training of a large cadre of research scientists who went on to show the power of equitable international partnerships.

Warren's influence continues to be felt in other institutions around the world. The Regius Professorship of Medicine at the University of Oxford, established in 1546, is the oldest scientific chair in England. When Sir David Weatherall was appointed to this prestigious post, he used it to advance our understanding of the mechanisms of disease. Through his ground-breaking work in thalassemia, a disease that disproportionately affects inhabitants of developing countries, Weatherall has helped thousands of children with this disease throughout the developing world. As the foundation leader of the Oxford GND group, he is in no doubt of the contribution that Warren's network made to the field of tropical medicine at Oxford: "the flexibility of the support was, to my mind, Ken Warren's major success. It enabled us to develop overseas links and to send people to carry out field work which would have been completely impossible under any other form of support. I only have to think of all our work in the Pacific Islands to realise how much we owed to the Rockefeller Foundation."[30] Such new opportunities were also realised in the founding of the Mahidol Oxford Tropical Medicine Research Unit in 1979, an innovation that had directly arisen from the inaugural meeting of the GND held in the previous year. Initially under the directorship of David Warrell and later Nick White, a major programme in malaria research was set up that has attracted outstanding scientists from Thailand, Vietnam, and across the world. The KEMRI Wellcome Trust Research Programme was established in 1989 in Kilifi on the east coast of Kenya. Its first director was Kevin Marsh, who has a broad interest in the clinical, epidemiological, and immunological aspects of malaria and in training a generation of African scientists in the state-of-the-art-laboratory in Kilifi. Serendipitously, Marsh had attended the final GND meeting, held at Taita Hills Wildlife Sanctuary in Kenya. It marked a profound moment which was to shape the future of Marsh's career: "I met Ken Warren a few times, but didn't know him well. Funnily, it was attending one of the network meetings in Kenya in 1987 that I ended up going down for the weekend to Kilifi… and the die was cast!"[31] Today, research into infectious diseases is performed at three Wellcome Trust Major Overseas Programmes in Kenya, Thailand, and Vietnam, together with a number of sister groups in Laos, Tanzania, Indonesia, and Nepal, as well as the Tropical Research Programme in Oxford (Fig. 6.4).

Likewise, at the Karolinska Institute in Sweden, Hans Wigzell and Peter Perlmann, funded by the GND, trained many young scientists, including Mats Wahlgren, who continue to work on the mechanisms of severe malaria. Warren also supported the outstanding work of the immunologist John David at The Harvard School of Public Health, who discovered the first cytokine MIF. Under David's

---

[30]David Weatherall, personal communication.

[31]Kevin Marsh, personal communication.

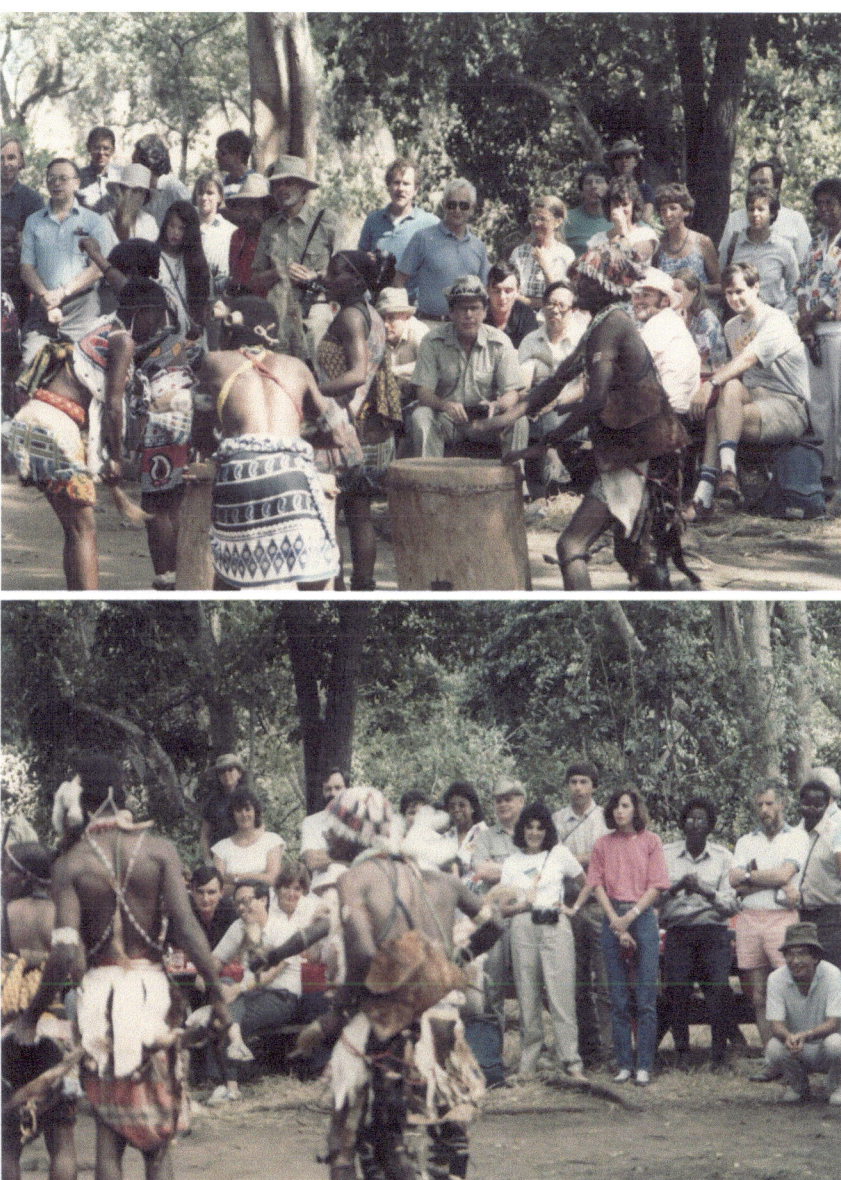

Fig. 6.4 Final GND meeting 1987, Taita Hills, Kenya. The meeting took place, at Ken's request, "under the snows of Mt Kilimanjaro". Top Photograph. Ken is in the centre of the photo wearing a green safari suit and hat, with John David just behind him, wearing sunglasses. Sylvia Warren is standing to John's left. Directly behind Sylvia, smoking a pipe, is Kevin Marsh, and standing on the extreme right of the image is Orneata Prawl. Second from left in a light blue shirt is Barry Bloom, and on the same row, three places to the right, is David Baltimore, in a red shirt and hat. Onesmo ole-MoiYoi is in the lower photograph, fourth from the right. Courtesy of Onesmo ole-MoiYoi

direction, many young scientists subsequently performed field research in the tropics.[32] Indeed, Warren's former group at Case Western Reserve University went on to become a strong force in malaria field research in Africa and Papua New Guinea.[33] Louis Miller, who was asked by Ken Warren to give the lecture on malaria at the first GND meeting held at the Abby Aldrich Rockefeller Hall in 1978, is in no doubt of his friend's contribution to parasitology: "It is only through research that the complex problems of parasitic diseases can be solved. Ken's legacy is the continuation of research at the highest level, with the bar set high by Ken himself. We are living his vision today."[34]

Warren's achievements contributed to the metamorphosis of parasitology during his lifetime. Possessing a linguistic talent for taxonomy, he invented a new vocabulary with the Great Neglected Diseases of Mankind Programme, which marked a semantic breakthrough in the evolution of what has become known as "global health." He influenced many of the individuals who have helped to define health priorities for global populations: Dean Jamison, Richard Peto, and Christopher Murray all recognise the wisdom of his approach, of his emphasis on the necessity of having good evidence, and of evaluating which health interventions, both in developed and developing countries, would be worthwhile in terms of benefit. Indeed, the concept of the inequity caused by global patterns of health inequality, and the emergence of the DALY as a metric of ill-health beyond mortality statistics, can both be traced back to Warren. Rather like Peto, Warren took a numerical view of international health aligned to the theory of cost-effectiveness. As a renowned advocate of large-scale randomised evidence and large-scale implementation, Peto recognises Warren's enduring contribution: "He influenced a great many ideas that we take for granted today. It is much more widely accepted now that his attitude, the Warren sort of attitude, is right...."[35]

Indeed, although many of the diseases targeted by the GND Programme continue to afflict the world's poorest people—there is still no fully effective vaccine against malaria for instance—prospects for reducing the health burden caused by neglected tropical diseases have become more favourable with the implementation of the five health-related aims of the United Nations Millennium Development Goals (MDGs). One of these, relating to the interplay between infection and malnutrition, has become the research focus for Onesmo ole-MoiYoi.[36] Onesmo's first encounter with Warren was in 1977 when he attended a lecture on tropical diseases

---

[32]Louis H. Miller, personal communication.

[33]A. E. Dent, R. Nakajimo, L. Liang, E. Baum, A. M. Moorman, P. Odada Sumba, J. Vulule, D. Banineau, D. Huw Davies, P. L. Felgner & J. W. Kazura, "*Plasmodium falciparum* Protein Microarray Antibody Profiles Correlate with Protection from Symptomatic Malaria in Kenya." J Infect Dis. 2015, 212 (9): 1429–1438.

[34]Louis H. Miller, personal communication.

[35]Richard Peto, personal communication.

[36]O. K. ole-MoiYoi, *Short-and Long-term Effects of Drought on Human Health*. Case Study prepared for the Global Assessment Report on Disaster Risk Reduction 2013. Geneva, Switzerland, 2013, pp. 1–30.

at Harvard: "I identified with him because we both went to Harvard and then Harvard Medical School. Ken was a warm person. I felt a connection both educationally and in the shared interest in tropical diseases, and the fact that he was looking at these diseases that affected 70% of the world's population, and that they were neglected … and not considered relevant. Ken brought attention to them by being provocative in a nice way."[37] The young scientist became interested in malnutrition while attending a GND seminar on growth stunting, in which evidence was presented that children were more susceptible to diseases depending upon which trimester food intake is at its most restricted before birth. Onesmo's research now focuses on ensuring that pregnant women have enough of the right food to eat as the immune system of children is compromised by malnutrition. In his own words, "Ken set me on this path."[38]

If Warren were alive today, he would almost certainly still be working on NTDs, but perhaps he would make greater efforts to ensure that more people in developing countries were doing the work. Steve Meshnick worked as a parasitologist in Kenya in the 1980s and recognises that more progress needs to be made: "The bottom line is that the people who want to get rid of these diseases are the people in the countries where the diseases are endemic … what you really need is a cadre of trained people in the developing countries who can do that. There have been efforts to do this, but it could be better."[39] Although the GND project established partnerships that had the potential to create this cohort of new scientists, it left much still to be done. Nevertheless, in recognition of Warren's important support of scientists in the developing world, and his advocacy of the free dissemination of evidence-based health research in those geographies, the Cochrane Collaboration established The Kenneth Warren Prize in 2000 to celebrate Warren's ideals.[40] The prize of $1000 is awarded annually to the principal author, who must be a national living in a developing country, of a published Cochrane Review that is judged to be both of high methodological quality and relevant to health problems in developing countries.

Warren believed that prevention was better than cure, and at the second Bellagio Conference he quoted his colleague, the immunologist Geoffrey Edsall: "Never in the history of human progress has a better and cheaper method of preventing illness been developed than immunisation at its best."[41] Undeniably the world of vaccine

---

[37]Onesmo ole-MoiYoi, personal communication.

[38]Onesmo ole-MoiYoi, personal communication.

[39]Steve Meshnick, personal communication.

[40]Ken Warren donated $10,000 to the fledgling Cochrane Collaboration, and in an act of financial symmetry, Sir Iain Chalmers donated $10,000 to the fund that established the Warren Prize. Among other individual and institutional donors were Eugene Garfield, Joe and Betty-Anne Cook, Phyllis Freeman and Anthony Robbins, and The Rockefeller Foundation.

[41]J. P. Grant, Address to the New York Academy of Sciences L.S. Frohlich Award Conference New York 18 October 1988. UNICEF publication, p. 6. Courtesy of Sylvia Warren.

development is highly complex, and one of the reasons why Warren was so dedicated to vaccines was that there were no safe drugs—in the era before praziquantel—with which to treat schistosomiasis. And there still has been no success with efforts to develop vaccines against human helminths. Nonetheless, by establishing the idea of the power and possibilities of biomedical science, nowhere more so than his faith in vaccines, Warren helped to nurture a generation of physician–scientists who have made prodigious contributions to a better understanding of human biology in both health and disease. The people he selected and the scientific attitude he embodied played an important role in establishing the scientific bedrock that underpins today's goal of translating research from the laboratory to the clinic. Whereas researchers had been looking for vaccines and other preventative measures against infectious diseases for many decades, it was Warren, by focusing on the need to find vaccines specifically against the GNDs, who helped to signpost the scientific way forward for today's leaders in global health.

One person at the forefront of infectious disease research is Jeremy Farrar, Director of the Wellcome Trust. He came to the post after working for 17 years as the head of Oxford's Wellcome-funded Clinical Research Unit in Ho Chi Minh City, Vietnam, which in part had been funded initially by the GND. Farrar forms a celebrated historical link with Peter Williams and Bridget Ogilvie, past directors of the Wellcome Trust, who were also dedicated to funding research into the infectious diseases that predominate in poorer regions of the world. In an article on 3 August 2015, Farrar, while writing about the spectacular success of the rVSV-ZEBOV vaccine in communities in patients with Ebola, made an appeal that was Warren-like in sentiment: "It is clear to me that what we urgently need now is a global vaccine development fund, with contributions from governments, philanthropic foundations and industry."[42] Vaccine research continues to be one of the most apposite topics of our time in the health field. In January 2015, at a major vaccine-funding conference in Berlin, Bill Gates praised companies investing in vaccine research for poor countries. In an interview with *The Guardian* newspaper, he stated that immunisation "is the cheapest thing ever done in health."[43] Meanwhile, Gavi, The Global Alliance for Vaccines and Immunisation, states that half a billion children have been immunised through its support in the last 15 years and that 7 million lives have been saved.[44]

In a pioneering article in 1990, Warren advocated a policy of mass drug administration that he believed would lead the beginning of the end of the diseases that had been the scourge of neglected people.[45] The intellectual ascendancy of his

---

[42]J. Farrar, "The Ebola vaccine we dared to dream of is here," *The Guardian*, 3 August 2015.

[43]*The Guardian*, 28 January 2015.

[44]Gavi mission statement, http://www.gavi.org/about/mission/.

[45]Warren, K.S. An integrated system for the control of the major human helminth parasites. Acta Leidensia **59**: 433–442, 1990.

belief in the integrated application of broad-spectrum anthelmintics, given in low doses at prolonged intervals, and the effectiveness of selective primary health care, were vindicated by the formation of the African Programme for Onchocerciasis Control (APOC) in 1995. The success of the community-directed treatment programme has not only prevented onchocerciasis from causing blindness in people living on the continent, it has also provided the mass drug-administration template for the future of NTD control in Africa and in other geographical areas. The 20-year APOC programme (1995–2015) was an example of public–private partnerships of various sorts—nongovernmental development organisations in partnerships with endemic countries, the World Bank Trust Fund, the World Health Organisation, and above all of the donation by Merck and Co Inc. of ivermectin (brand name Mectizan), which made APOC possible. Dirk Engels, Director of the Department of Control of NTDs at the WHO, recognises the contribution that Warren has made to contemporary thinking. "Ken's idea of selective primary health care—that is where it all started. Ken and Julia Walsh did the groundwork, and APOC built upon it."[46]

The year 2015 proved to be an auspicious one for tropical diseases and immunisation. In addition to being the 15th anniversary of the creation of Gavi, the year also saw the Nobel Prize in Physiology or Medicine awarded to three scientists who developed therapies against parasitic infections. The winners were William C. Campbell, a microbiologist at Drew University in Madison, New Jersey; Satoshi Ōmura, a microbiologist at Kitasato University in Japan; and Youyou Tu, a pharmacologist at the China Academy of Chinese Medical Sciences in Beijing. In the 1970s, Campbell and Ōmura discovered a class of compounds, called avermectins, that kill the parasitic roundworms that cause infections such as river blindness and lymphatic filariasis. The most potent of these was released onto the market in 1981 as the drug ivermectin. Tu developed the antimalarial drug artemisinin in the late 1960s and 1970s. These outstanding scientists used modern laboratory techniques to discover anti-parasitic drugs. The award of the Nobel Prize to these scientists highlights the importance of parasitic infections and neglected tropical diseases and builds on the efforts of the Gates Foundation to elevate NTDs in the public's mind. Yet although there may be a renaissance of interest, there is still a perception that NTDs are not well understood in the richer countries of the world at the political and social level.[47] The explanation may in part be because the fascinating story of neglected tropical diseases has not been well told in the history of medicine. This book brings Ken Warren's contribution to this remarkable story into sharper focus. His sacrifices and achievements continue to inform us in the present era, and his strategies to ameliorate the unsolved problems of disease control in efficient,

---

[46]Dirk Engels, personal communication.
[47]Don Bundy, personal communication.

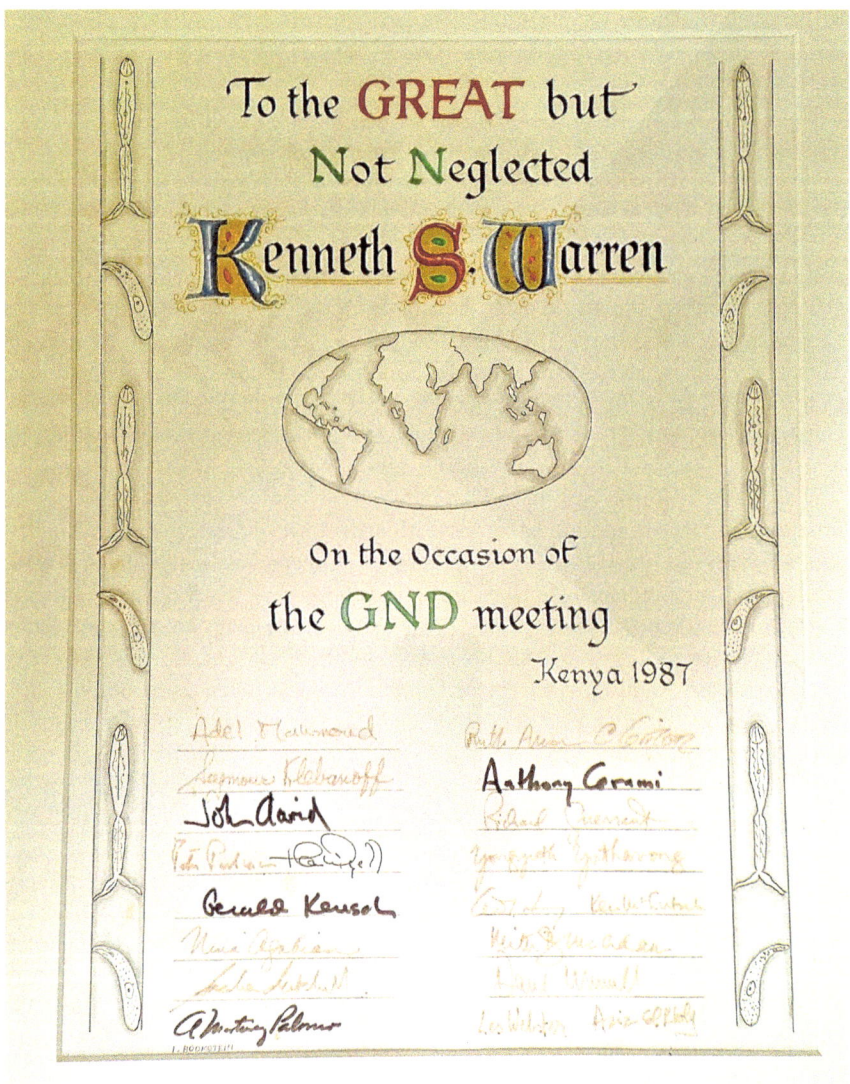

Fig. 6.5 This degree certificate was presented to Warren by his GND colleagues at the end of the final GND meeting, 1987. Courtesy of Erica Warren

creative, and practical ways are a vindication of his life's work. In light of his continued relevance to the field of neglected tropical diseases and global health, this book should not be the last word on Warren: a prescient, influential, and highly complex "tropical medicine man" (Fig. 6.5).

Index

© Springer International Publishing AG 2017
C. Keating, *Kenneth Warren and the Great Neglected Diseases of Mankind Programme*, Springer Biographies,
DOI 10.1007/978-3-319-50147-5